THE NICU ROLLERCOASTER

Salem Hospital Library
Discarded
Note: May contain outdated information!

Please return to:
**Salem Health
Community Health Education Center**
939 Oak Street SE, Building D • Salem, OR 97301
Phone: 503-814-2432 or 1-866-977-2432
Email: CHEC@salemhospital.org
Web: www.salemhealth.org/chec

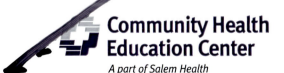

Community Health Education Center
A part of Salem Health

The NICU Rollercoaster

How to Set Up and Use an Online Blog to Help Survive the Ups, Downs, Agonies, and Joys of Your Baby's Stay

Nicole E. Zimmerman
and
Edward J. Sprague

Copyright © 2008 by Nicole E. Zimmerman and Edward J. Sprague.

Front cover photograph and author photographs by Aimee Bickers, Pure Expressions Photography, Apex, NC

Library of Congress Control Number: 2008904691
ISBN: Hardcover   978-1-4363-2655-1
       Softcover   978-1-4363-2654-4

All rights reserved. No part of this book may be reproduced or transmitted in any form or by any means, electronic or mechanical, including photocopying, recording, or by any information storage and retrieval system, without permission in writing from the copyright owner.

This book was printed in the United States of America.

To order additional copies of this book, contact:
Xlibris Corporation
1-888-795-4274
www.Xlibris.com
Orders@Xlibris.com

Contents

Acknowledgments 9
Authors' Notes 11
Introduction 15

Part 1   The Ride Begins 17
Part 2   Riding the Rollercoaster 43
Part 3   Adjusting with Setbacks 107
Part 4   Reality Check: The Ride Does Not Ever End,
             But the Rewards Are Enormous 149

Epilogue 175
References 177
Author's Biography 179

DEDICATION

For our children, Ronan and Julia. You have come so far and grown so much. We are thankful to have you here with us.

Acknowledgments

Ed and I will be forever grateful to the North Carolina Children's Hospital in Chapel Hill, North Carolina. Without the medical expertise and compassionate care provided by the staff, this story would have had a different ending. In particular, we'd like to thank Amy, Dawn, Elizabeth, Dr. Wood, and our rocks, Aimee and Amber. We would also like to thank our family, friends, and loyal CarePages readers and contributors for their support from July 7, 2006, through the present.

Authors' Notes

We have pledged 25 percent of the royalties of the sale of this book, to be provided to the March of Dimes.

This book is simply meant to tell our story and give guidance to other NICU parents about what to expect after giving birth to a premature infant. However, it is not intended to provide medical advice, diagnosis, or treatment. Always talk to your physician or other qualified health provider with any questions you may have regarding your infant's prematurity.

The March of Dimes wishes to thank the authors for helping to increase awareness of the seriousness of premature birth and the realities of life in the NICU.

The sole focus of the March of Dimes is the health of all babies, those born healthy and those who need support to survive and thrive. Since our founding in 1938 we have invested in Nobel Prize-winning research to find solutions to problems that threaten infant health including both premature birth and birth defects. Over the years, March of Dimes advances such as neonatal intensive care units, newborn screening tests, and genetic therapies, have saved the lives and health of millions of babies.

Today, our top priority is the problem of premature birth. Prematurity affects more than half a million babies and their families every year and the rate continues to rise. With everyone's support, we are funding all important research by the best scientists in order find ways to help more pregnancies go full term, educating families about risk factors and symptoms of preterm labor, and providing information and comfort to families with babies in neonatal intensive care through our NICU Family Support® program.

We'd like you to know about our wide variety of online resources that pregnant women and new families will find particularly helpful.

- **Shareyourstory.org**—A special online community for families of sick or premature babies. Here you can connect with others who've had similar experiences and who understand. Share your story, get information, and find emotional support.
- **Marchofdimes.com**—Our site is packed with vital health information for pregnant women and new moms.
- *Askus@marchofdimes.com*—If you don't find the information you need on our site or have a personal question, e-mail us and you'll get a personal answer from one of our health information specialists.
- **Podcasts**—A variety of pregnancy and newborn health topics are available for downloading or just listening.
- **Everybabyhasastory.org**—Our growing online community where you can tell your baby's special story and read thousands of others' stories.

Introduction

You are about to go on a journey that for some of us lasts three days, for others six months. Whether your child is in the neonatal intensive care unit (NICU) for a short period of time or a long period of time, it is an agonizing journey. Some of us battled with infertility and were finally able to conceive only to learn that we were having multiples. Others of us had more typical pregnancies until something went wrong. All types of couples with endless varieties of situations can end up in the NICU.

We met parents in the NICU with full-term babies who had medical complications; parents of triplets where only one survived; parents of twins with twin-to-twin transfusion—a condition where one baby does not get enough nutrition and does not grow as fast as the other baby; parents of single babies born at twenty-four weeks; parents of babies who did not make it; and many parents like us who had long stays in the NICU but eventually got to take their babies home.

Whatever your circumstances, you are going to need some emotional support and a plan to follow to get through possibly the hardest thing you've had to face. Many parents will have happy endings and some will not, but either way it is going to take a lot of personal strength and support from your loved ones and even from strangers to get through this.

This book will provide tips on how to survive the NICU from the day of your baby's birth until the day your baby comes home. Tips offered include:

- How to deal with the guilt you may feel at having a premature baby;
- How to take advantage of offers from your friends and loved ones to help without getting overwhelmed;
- How to use a blog to help improve communication, decrease stress, and keep everyone informed;
- How to deal with the financial aspects of having a baby in the NICU;
- How to adjust to daily life when your baby finally comes home.

We plan to attend the next NICU reunion at our hospital to see how all of the former twenty-four, twenty-five, twenty-six, and twenty-seven+ weekers fared. We heard that the reunion is always packed with happy parents and kids, many of whom bear few scars emotionally or physically from their stays in the NICU.

Part 1

The Ride Begins

Whether you have had a difficult pregnancy or your premature baby is a complete surprise, the day you board the NICU rollercoaster will be emotionally trying. On the day of my twins' birth, the surgeon took my husband aside and told him there was probably only a 50 percent chance they would live. He didn't tell me this until several months later. I'm glad he didn't tell me, but I feel terrible that he had to bear news like that on his own.

My husband Ed and I had been trying to have a child for two years. We started when I was thirty-three. We conceived about a year later with the help of fertility drugs. I had an early miscarriage at seven weeks, but within another year, I conceived twins. Yes, twins—it can happen to anyone. Double the fun. Double the trouble. We heard it all, and we were nervous. In the first trimester, I was worried about miscarriage, birth defects and hoping they'd be healthy, my not feeling well and how and when to tell the boss. In the second trimester, I was worried about the potential of being put on bed rest, how big I was going to get in the third trimester, and working out a leave of absence plan for work. But everything was going well. Every time I went to the doctor, he was happy with my weight and the progress of the babies on the ultrasounds.

I started off reading a lot. I had the typical *What to Expect When You Are Expecting* book. I also had a book on twins, and I had the Internet. I found that the Internet is not a good place to go for someone who is expecting and is nervous about it. I read about things that no one should ever read about. Being a type A personality, I tried to get an A in pregnancy. I took my vitamins, ate a balanced diet, exercised, avoided alcohol, secondhand smoke, and chemicals. The only thing I got a B in was controlling stress, but that particular item was very difficult for me to control. I did feel a lot better after I passed the twelve-week mark without incident, and nothing out of the ordinary showed up on the prenatal tests for birth defects.

We took a trip up the East Coast during my twenty-fourth week of pregnancy to see our families and have a baby shower. We returned home late in the afternoon on Wednesday, July 5. On Friday morning, July 7, Ed and I went to the OB/GYN at 8:00 a.m. for my monthly appointment. We were always nervous before these appointments. We never knew what we were going to see on the ultrasound, and we hoped that everything would be OK. The ultrasound went fine. The babies were both growing the way they were supposed to grow. The ultrasound technician said, "Julia is kicking Ronan in the head and quarters are about to get very tight."

Next I went in to see one of the OB/GYN doctors. She was one I had not seen before. There are several doctors in the practice, so the patients need to meet each doctor at least once before they deliver. She asked me some questions, did an exam, and then asked for my questions. I asked, "Is it OK if I keep exercising, and is it OK for me to paint the nursery?" She smiled as she answered, "Everything is going as planned, and I'm pleased with your progress, Nicole. I do want to check your cervix for a baseline before you leave, though." She did her exam, and all of a sudden, the atmosphere in the room changed.

She looked a lot more serious and said, "I can feel your bag of waters bulging, and the cervix has started to dilate. This is concerning to me." She talked about hospitalization and bed rest and trying to keep the babies in the womb. This was the first time of many to follow that I would hear a doctor use the phrase "concerning to me."

"I'm going to leave the room now and give you and Ed some time to absorb what I've said," she told us.

I was so scared. I was more scared than I had ever been in my whole life. Why was this happening? It was too early. We had fifteen more weeks to go. How could we have the babies now? They weren't ready to enter the world. It was an unreal moment that is frozen in my brain. The room appeared very bright and sterile, and Ed hugged me after the doctor had left. We both cried.

After awhile she came back and said she was admitting me to the hospital. She put me in a wheelchair and wheeled me over to the hospital. They took me straight up to the maternity ward. The nurse allowed me to go to the bathroom and then had me change into a hospital gown and lie in a hospital bed.

How could this happen? Friday, July 7, was just a normal day in a normal life, but now everything was turned upside down. They put all sorts of monitoring equipment on me and raised my feet so that the babies would stay in. They gave me an IV with medicine to try to stop the labor. The labor? How could I be in labor? None of this made sense. It was way too early. They also gave me a shot that would help the babies' lungs if they couldn't stop the labor. They said the longer they could keep them in, the better off the lungs would be. Ed left to call our parents and the nurse left the room.

The NICU Rollercoaster

I was all alone to think about what was happening. The hours passed, and the nurses and doctors came in and out. One doctor said, "We can't keep you here. We need to get you over to Duke or UNC Hospital where they'll be able to take care of the babies. The NICU here is not equipped to take care of twenty-five weekers." I lay there for several hours and tried to deny the inevitable. I was in labor.

I started to feel uncomfortable at regular intervals but would not admit to myself what was happening. Then fluid seemed to come out every time I felt uncomfortable. I thought I was losing control of my bladder. I am surprised even today at the level of denial I was in. Finally one of the nurses said that it wasn't urine; it was likely amniotic fluid. My water was breaking. They checked my cervix again and saw it had not gotten any larger. "Maybe we can stop your labor, but you have months of bed rest ahead of you," the doctor concluded.

I had always said that there was no way anyone could confine me to bed. I would go nuts. It seemed like a joke. I would outwit them and not have to go on bed rest. But over the hours I lay there, the picture started to change for me. I began to understand why the doctor would order that, and it seemed like a really good idea. A doctor explained that, "Every hour we can keep the babies in will help them. Even if it is only a few days, it'll be enough time for their lungs to mature a little more. Time is our friend in this."

I was told that they were going to transport me to UNC Hospitals. They have a level three neonatal intensive care unit that can handle twenty-five-week-old infants. Apparently, twenty-five weeks is close to the cutoff point for human life. These days, a twenty-five weeker is probably going to make it, but an extra week can really make a difference. Twenty-three and twenty-four weekers are much more iffy.

Two EMTs came into my room in flight suits, carrying a stretcher. They also handle the helicopter transports, but thankfully, I was going in the ambulance. Not that I wouldn't enjoy a helicopter ride under different circumstances. As they rolled me out, I saw people looking at me in the hallways probably wondering what was wrong with me. That is what I wonder when I see someone on a stretcher.

The ride to the hospital took forever. One of the EMTs drove and the other stayed in the back with me. I could see the tops of the trees going by out the high windows of the ambulance. The EMT looked at my charts a lot and took my vitals. After we arrived at the hospital, they wheeled me in a back entrance and into a room with a big window looking out over Chapel Hill.

A fantastic nurse there, Jennifer, seemed to understand how scared I was, and somehow she made me feel better. A few minutes later, Ed walked in. He had followed us to the hospital in our car. At this point, it seemed that they would be able to hold off my labor for a while.

But things soon turned. The resident cheerfully told me, "Nicole, you have dilated to five centimeters. The babies are so tiny that we can't keep them in. To make things more interesting, Julia is in breech position so we'll have to do a C-section and soon." This was a very bad dream. For weeks afterward, I kept thinking I might wake up, everything would be fine, and none of this would have happened.

They wheeled me over to the operating room, which was as bright and sterile as the earlier one. A lot of people were milling around—residents, interns, nurses, pediatricians, surgeons, students, and on and on. There were probably twenty-five people in the room. Preparation for the surgery seemed to go on for a long time. They sat me up and gave me a spinal block in my back. It felt so strange. Jennifer stayed with me the whole time and gave me a hug as they did the spinal block. She did a great job keeping me calm. Eventually Ed came in, and they put a big blanket up, and it was time to deliver the twins.

I started shaking, and one of the doctors asked, "Are you cold?" "I'm not sure. I think I'm cold or scared or both."

"Well, it's normal. In any case, shaking and shivering are just side effects of the medication." Still, I was nervous that I would jerk at the wrong moment, and they would cut the wrong place.

The C-section seemed to take a long time. At one point, Ed peeked over the curtain and described how he saw all my insides lying on my stomach. I couldn't see him because they took my glasses, but I'll bet at that point he looked a little pale.

Julia came out first at 5:13 p.m., but they didn't show her to me like they do on television. They just scooped her out and rushed her out of the room since it wasn't big enough for me and two babies and all the medical staff.

Ronan came out less than a minute later. They took him over to a corner of the room and started to work on him. I didn't get a real good view, but I heard him cry before they inserted a breathing tube or, as they say, "intubated" him. They let Ed go over to the next room and see Julia while they finished up with me. It didn't hurt, but I felt a lot of pressure on my abdomen. They seemed to take longer to put me back together than it took to get the babies out.

They rolled me down to recovery, and it seemed as though I was there for a long time. A woman next to us was screaming and had to go into surgery without a spinal block because the baby was coming so quickly. When she woke up, she was in a lot of pain. Nurse Jennifer came and spent some time with me. Finally it was time to move to my room. Ed went to call people, and I don't really remember what I was doing. I knew I wanted to see the kids, but the NICU staff was still working on them.

The hours ticked by and around 10:00 p.m. I demanded to see the kids. The nurse said she was waiting for one of the doctors to write a pain prescription for me, and everyone was busy. I chose to go anyway. I was not going to wait any longer. It might not have been the smartest decision. Every bump on the way down—moving from carpet to hard floor, going into the elevator—hurt beyond belief. They rolled me into Pod B where we were to spend many, many weeks.

Our hospital had a wonderful resource that the staff encouraged us to use. When patients are faced with a long or tough hospitalization, the hospital offers the use of a blogging or e-diary service. Here is my first e-entry to the blog:

1 July 16, 2006

Julia Rachel Sprague and Ronan Bradley Sprague were born at 5:13 p.m. on July 7, 2006. Julia weighed 1 lb 9 oz. Ronan weighed 2 lbs 2 oz. They were born at twenty-five weeks and two days. It was a big surprise for us—the pregnancy was going well, but a routine visit to the OB/GYN Friday morning turned scary when the doctor discovered that I had started to go into labor. They tried to stop the labor but failed. They transported me to UNC which has an excellent neonatal intensive care unit, and the twins were born that evening.

*** *Typical first impressions of the NICU*

- Is that tiny little person really my baby?
- Why are there so many tubes and machines hooked up to my baby?
- Even though she only weighs a pound and a half, she still has all of her parts—a nose, a mouth, two arms, two legs, two hands, two feet, and ten fingers and ten toes.
- Is he going to make it?

Our first glimpse of them was intimidating. They were lying in big beds with a clear tent over them and blue lights shining down on them. I later found out that the tents were to keep their tender new skin moist and the lights were to control their bilirubin levels. They were so tiny and red, and there were tubes sticking out everywhere. They both seemed to have all their limbs, fingers, and toes and their features were perfect miniatures of full-term babies. However, both babies still had their eyelids fused together, which is common in premature babies. The nurse for my room came down and gave me the long-awaited painkillers, and everything else was a little fuzzy after that. I don't think we stayed too long. I was suddenly very tired.

Whether you are recovering from a vaginal birth or a C-section, now is the time to learn how the NICU works.

*** *Life in the NICU*

- When the doctor says your baby will probably not go home until at least her due date, believe her. When our twins were born at twenty-five weeks,

forty weeks seemed like a lifetime away, and we both harbored a secret fantasy that they'd be able to come home earlier.
- Participate in the care of your baby.
  o Ask the nurses if you can change the baby or take his temperature.
  o Nursing or pumping is one of the most important things you can do to improve your baby's chances for survival. Even if you only get a few drops, it will help your baby.
  o If your baby is too small to nurse, ask the nurses if your hospital has lactation consultants. The lactation consultants can help you find the right equipment and teach you how to pump.
  o If your baby is healthy enough, ask whether you can hold her.
- Communication is key.
  o Ask your nurse for an update each day.
  o Ask to speak to the nurse practitioner or attending physician to discuss short-term and long-term goals for your baby.
  o In short, learn as much as you can by asking the nurses and physicians lots of questions.
  o Keep a notepad and pencil nearby so you can jot down questions as you think of them.
  o If your NICU has a parents' room, take advantage of the library and/or Internet to get more information on the topics that are important to you.
  o Read, but not too much. If your child has a problem, read about it. However, don't look up every problem that a preemie could have, or you could drive yourself crazy.

I stayed in the hospital for four days and went down to see the twins several times each day. I spent a lot of time reliving that last week and trying to figure out what I did wrong. Should we not have traveled up to New York? Should we have skipped the afternoon shopping? Should I have gone to the hospital Thursday night when I didn't feel right? I never felt good when I was pregnant, so how was I supposed to know what was normal and what was not?

*** *How to deal with the guilt*

- Don't blame yourself. Don't analyze every minute of every week of your pregnancy trying to pinpoint what you did wrong to cause the baby to come early. In most cases the cause is unknown and/or out of your control. It is better to focus on the present.
- Find your inner strength. It sounds like a sappy saying you'd read on one of those framed posters they hang up in office hallways. But this is

a good exercise for growing up and learning what you are made of. You'd be surprised how much you can handle when there isn't any other choice. Fortunately, there is an enticing prize at the end of the road—taking your baby home.

I was excited to go home, but sad too. I started to cry as we left the hospital. I never, in a million years, pictured leaving our babies at the hospital. All of things I had worried about during the pregnancy suddenly seemed very silly. For some reason, premature birth never occurred to me.

The first week home was really hard. I was pumping around the clock and traveling back and forth to the hospital. It was all very overwhelming and exhausting. The worst part was that there was no end in sight. We'd be going back and forth to the hospital every day for months on end. We were told Julia and Ronan would likely stay in the hospital until their original due date of October 18, 2006, or longer, depending on how things progressed. At this point they couldn't tell us about their long-term prognosis. In fact, it could be years before we found out whether our twins will suffer any long-term effects from their very early appearance in the world. In the early days, I worried a lot about what long-term issues they would have. As they get older, I am not quite so focused on that. I try to focus on their day-to-day progress instead.

*** *NICU Tips*

- When parents refer to the NICU as a rollercoaster, it is an accurate description. The first few days after the baby is born are called the honeymoon period. Around the sixth or seventh day, your baby tends to have his first dip. After that, the ups and downs keep coming.
- Primary care nurses will help you get through your ordeal. Each infant in our NICU had two primary care nurses. The primary nurse cares for her primary baby every day she is at work. Because she knows the baby so well, she helps manage and direct the care. She becomes the baby's advocate to make sure that she gets the best care possible. The primary nurse also forms a relationship with the parents to help them feel more comfortable with their premature baby and teach them the lay of the NICU.
- Breastfeeding isn't fun when you have to do it by machine. Preemies are not generally able to take a bottle or breastfeed until about thirty-five weeks. If you want to breastfeed, you need to pump milk for them until they are ready to suck. Even if you can only pump a little, it will help him a lot.
- Everyone cares. It is amazing how much support you'll both get from people you know well and people you don't know so well.

- Some people have an "instinct" for what to do that is most helpful. Some people don't have it. The most helpful friend or relative is the one that anticipates your needs and takes care of them. When someone offers to help, you can be overwhelmed with trying to figure out what he/she can help with. When someone does something helpful without asking, it can be a huge load off your back. Figure out who's who and keep the most helpful nearby for support.
- Here are some things that friends and family did that were very helpful:
  - When we unexpectedly ended up in the hospital after a routine doctor's appointment, we did not have our "packed suitcase" for the hospital. In fact, we didn't have anything. At week twenty-five we weren't even thinking about packing a suitcase for the hospital. One of our good friends showed up at the hospital at nine o'clock that night with a bag, including a change of clothes, a hair band, snacks, socks, reading material, lotion, sanitary wipes, lip balm, toiletries, nursing bras, and breast pads for leaking. That was probably the most thoughtful thing anyone has ever done for us.
  - The same friend also called another friend who had NICU experience. She arranged for her to come see the babies and talk us through things. She didn't ask us to make any decisions. She just informed us when our friend would arrive. Our friend spent several hours with us and explained how things worked in the NICU. She basically talked us down off the ceiling. It is amazing how some people just know the right things to do and say. It is quite a gift.
  - We left a key hidden in the yard. Our friends came by to mow, clean, assemble baby furniture, and deliver meals. When your babies are fighting for life, these are things you don't want to think about.
  - Some friends brought fresh fruits and vegetables while I was in the hospital. Hospital food isn't necessarily very healthy, and when you are trying to produce milk, you need to eat healthy, nutritious foods.
- Talking on the phone was overwhelming for us. We know all of our friends and family meant well when calling and leaving messages. However, this was an overly emotional experience, and it is difficult to describe it to caller after caller without breaking down. We wanted to return all the phone calls, but for the first few weeks, we didn't feel like doing a lot of talking.
- The hospital offered a service called CarePages. This allows you to set up a password-protected blog to give everyone daily or weekly updates on your situation. It is much easier to type one update than call many people and give it to them individually. It only took a few

minutes to set up and gave everyone the real-time information they were seeking.
- CarePages.com is an online community of support for people coping with a significant health issue. At CarePages.com, you can create your own personal CarePage—a free private, personalized Web page that allows you to share updates with family and friends, receive messages of encouragement and support, read stories and tips, and meet others in similar situations. Visit *www.CarePages.com* to get started!
- The CarePages made us feel better. We had a chance to express what we were feeling and try to make sense out of everything that was going on around us. The NICU had a parents' room, and we really looked forward to going in to enter our updates. The CarePages have a section where people can write messages. We also looked forward to reading the encouraging comments our friends and family wrote for us. If you are not computer literate, this is something someone can help with when they want to know what they can do to help.

2 July 17, 2006

The UNC Hospital neonatal intensive care unit (NICU) is divided into six pods or rooms. Each pod has between six and ten babies. The babies are cared for by specially trained NICU nurses around the clock. The nurses work from 7:00 a.m. to 7:30 p.m. and from 7:00 p.m. to 7:30 a.m. The overlapping half hours are spent "giving report" to the nurse coming on the new shift. We are allowed to visit anytime except twice a day, during report.

The nurses say that parents are part of the recovery, and we are encouraged to spend as much time with the babies as possible. The parents are even asked to become involved in the baby's care. We change diapers and take temperatures during care times. When they start feeding by bottle, we'll be encouraged to feed them as well. Right now, they are too little to feed by bottle or breast. Premature babies don't have their sucking mechanisms developed yet. The sucking, swallowing, and breathing pattern is something that even a full-term baby needs to learn to do. For now, they receive my breast milk through a feeding tube down their throats.

Julia's kidney function is not quite where it should be, but that is common in preemies, and they are watching it closely. They did an ultrasound of her brain today to check for bleeds, and everything looks OK. They also scanned her heart and determined that she has a patent ductus arteriosus or PDA. Before birth, the two major arteries are connected by a blood vessel called the ductus arteriosus. After birth, the vessel is supposed to close. In some babies, it remains open which can put a strain on the heart and increase the blood pressure in the lung arteries. They don't like to give medicine for the PDA when the kidneys aren't in an acceptable range, so they will watch her very closely in the next few days. She has been getting feedings and gained a little weight last night, which makes me feel a lot better.

We've gotten to hold Julia "kangaroo care" for about an hour each day, which makes Ed and me feel a lot better. During kangaroo care, the baby lies on her stomach on Mommy or Daddy's chest. A blanket is put over her back to create a pouch similar to a kangaroo pouch. The baby wears only a diaper, and Mom and Dad take off their tops so there is skin-to-skin contact. The baby is placed over the heart so she can hear a familiar sound she heard from the womb.

We're also told that she recognizes Mom's scent and Dad's voice. It is very comfortable for the baby and aids in healing and growing. Babies that are kangarooed tend to get discharged earlier than babies who are not held often. It is also very calming for the parents. Kangarooing is pretty much the only time we have felt relaxed since they were born. There is something about it that really calmed us down and helped us feel more optimistic.

During the first week of life, the doctors discovered that Ronan had a perforation in his bowel. In order to drain the fluids that had leaked into the abdomen, they inserted a Penrose drain in his belly. They are hoping that the perforation will heal itself and that surgery will not be necessary.

Necrotizing enterocolitis (NEC) is a disease that a premature baby can experience within the first weeks of life. "Necrotizing" means the death of tissue, "entero" refers to the small intestine, "colo" to the large intestine, and "itis" means inflammation.

NEC is a gastrointestinal disease that mostly affects premature infants. NEC involves infection and inflammation that causes destruction of the bowel or part of the bowel. Although it affects only one in two thousand to four thousand births, or between 1 percent and 5 percent of neonatal intensive care unit (NICU) admissions, NEC is the most common and serious gastrointestinal disorder among hospitalized preterm infants.

NEC typically occurs within the first two weeks of life, usually after milk feeding has begun (at first, feedings are usually given through a tube that goes directly to the baby's stomach). About 10 percent of babies weighing less than 1,500 grams (3 lbs 5 oz) experience NEC. These premature infants have immature bowels, which are sensitive to changes in blood flow and prone to infection. They may have difficulty with blood and oxygen circulation and digestion, which increases their chances of developing NEC.

In severe cases of NEC and in Ronan's case, a hole or perforation develops in the intestine, which can allow bacteria to leak into the abdomen, causing life-threatening infection called peritonitis. Because the infant's body systems are immature, even with quick treatment for NEC, there may be serious complications.

Because of the NEC, Ronan is not receiving any feedings or kangaroo care right now. He also has a large PDA, but they can't give him medicine because of the perforation and because he received high doses of blood pressure medication to control his blood pressure. They are hoping the perforation will heal itself, but they may have to do surgery later on to correct the PDA.

Our other concern with Ronan is bleeding in his brain or intraventricular hemorrhage. Dr. Patricia Bromberger, MD, a neonatologist at Kaiser Permanente states that an intraventricular hemorrhage (IVH) is a type of bleeding from fragile blood vessels in the brain. These blood vessels are especially fragile in premature infants. Babies born more than eight weeks early are most likely to have this bleeding.

Some fragile blood vessels surround the ventricles of the brain, cavities in the brain through which cerebrospinal fluid (CSF) flows. The blood vessels are underdeveloped in the very young infant. They start getting stronger after thirty-two weeks of gestation. These blood vessels are very sensitive to changes in blood flow. If the blood flow changes, the blood vessels break down and start bleeding. If the bleeding is slight, the blood remains around the blood vessels. If the bleeding gets worse, the blood breaks into the ventricles. In the worst cases of bleeding, the blood may leak into the brain tissue.

The hemorrhages are graded from 1 to 4 according to the severity of the bleeding. Small amounts of bleeding (grades 1 to 2) do not usually cause any long-term damage. Larger amounts of bleeding (grades 3 to 4) cause long-term problems. Grades 3 and 4 cause blood clots that can block the circulation system for the cerebrospinal fluid. This blockage is called hydrocephalus.

There is no test or examination that can accurately predict what a premature baby will be like as a child or adult. Only time and growth will show whether the brain has been permanently hurt.

Sometimes other parts of the baby's brain may be able to take over the function of any damaged areas. This means that babies often do much better than expected. They do much better than an adult with a similar brain injury. Love, care, and encouragement, which the child receives from his family, also have a very important effect on his outcome.

In general, babies who have had small amounts of bleeding (grades 1 and 2) do not have any more problems than other premature babies who did not have IVH. Babies who have had more severe bleeding are more likely to have developmental problems as they grow. Many children who have had a grade 4 hemorrhage may have problems controlling movement on the side of their body opposite that of the injured part of the brain. If the other side of the brain is normal, these children can often function well enough to attend regular school. Only time will tell to what extent a child's brain is injured and what long-term problems he will have.

When they did Ronan's initial cranial ultrasound scan, they found a grade 1 bleed on one side and a grade 4 bleed on the other. Needless to say, we were very upset after the doctor explained the implications of the bleeds. After waiting a week, they did a follow-up cranial ultrasound to see if the bleeding had gotten worse. Upon closer examination of the ultrasound, his doctors saw that Ronan had a grade 1 bleed on one side and a grade 2 bleed on the other. The difference between a grade 2 and a grade 4 bleed is tremendous in its long-term implications. In addition, the bleeding did not appear to have gotten any worse on the second ultrasound. This was one of the better pieces of news we received about Ronan since he arrived. They would do a final ultrasound before Ronan left the hospital.

3 July 18, 2006

Today the twins are eleven days old. They both had a good night. The doctors scanned Ronan's head and found that there was little change in the bleeding, which is very good news. They are also happy with the work that the Penrose drain is doing and think the perforation in his intestine may heal without the need for surgery.

Julia gained forty-three grams last night. A baby this size should gain ten to fifteen grams each day. The large weight gain could be a result of variations caused by the time they weighed her, the scale they used, and whether they adjusted for the weight of the diaper. Odds are that she may lose a few grams in the next couple of days. They have increased her feedings from 1 ml to 2 ml, and she seems to be tolerating them well.

I was able to kangaroo with Julia again today. I read in one of the preemie magazines that kangaroo care originated in Columbia where there was little access to reliable power or equipment. Despite these limitations, implementing kangaroo care decreased the mortality rate of premature infants significantly.

She really seems to enjoy her time with me, and I know I enjoy my time with her. I can't wait until Ronan is able to kangaroo again. I'd really like for Ed to try it too.

CarePages has a section where family and friends can leave messages of encouragement. This is one of our favorite parts of having the CarePage. On a bad day, a couple of notes from friends or family can really make a difference. We really appreciate everyone's emotional support.

Always in our thoughts!

July 18, 2006, at 10:29 PM EDT

Thank you so much for setting this up. I have bookmarked the page for future use! We are keeping you guys in our thoughts and prayers and have our church's

prayer team on the job too. As you know, we're always here for you if you need us—any time of day.
Hang in there!

((hugs))
Aimee and family

Week 27

4 July 19, 2006

Julia has gained another thirty grams. She is devouring all of the mother's milk she is given and is starting to add some fat to her skin and bones. She keeps the nurses on their toes with the large leak she has in her ventilator.

Ronan had a bit of a setback. His blood pressure dropped, and he was placed back on blood pressure medication. This afternoon they were able to turn it down again. They were concerned about his liver, but so far, it looks good. The hole in his intestine continues to heal. Another day has finally come to a close. Let's hope for a good Thursday.

Sounds like a good day!

July 19, 2006, at 09:50 PM EDT

I want to encourage you guys to get over to the NICU forum on Twinstuff. I was reading today about a set of twins born at twenty-six weeks who also dealt with brain bleeds and other issues you have told me about, and they are now healthy and happy two year olds! So your time will come, hang in there! We are always thinking about you, guys!

Aimee

Love from Tokyo

July 19, 2006, at 12:18 PM EDT

Hello Nicole, Ed, Ronan, and Julia
Wishing all four of you a lot of strength. Praying for a little more robustness and weight gain every day—one gram or forty-five grams at a time. Keep the faith and try to do something celebratory every twenty-four hours.

Love, Uncle Justin

5 July 20, 2006

Today Ronan's weight has gone up and Julia's has come down. Sometimes they lose weight after they've had a few days of gaining weight. They've increased Julia's feedings to 5 ml—I'm having trouble keeping up.

They are concerned about Julia's PDA and will start giving her some medicine called Indocin tomorrow to correct the problem. They have a few tests remaining before they can make the final call. They just want to make sure all her levels are acceptable before they start it. She will have a three-day course of Indocin, but they will have to stop her feedings during this time. However, we believe it is well worth it if it corrects the PDA. They are even talking about possibly removing her ventilator tube (or extubating her) next week if all goes well. That would be fantastic if she can tolerate it since the leak is still causing a problem. However, we know we have to take one thing at a time.

They are very happy with the progress on Ronan's drain. They may be able to remove it in a few days, and we hope this means that the hole in the intestine will heal itself without having to repair it surgically. He is still on blood pressure medicine including the hydrocortisone, so he is not a candidate for Indocin to fix his PDA. Right now they are concerned about his bilirubin levels. They are not where they should be, and they are not sure why. So far, most of the tests results have been in the acceptable range. They think it might be caused by a fungal infection so they are going to start antibiotics to correct it.

We love you guys

July 20, 2006, at 06:59 PM EDT

Ed, Nicole, Ronan, and Julia: We are thinking about all four of you all of the time, and you are in our prayers. One day at a time. We can't wait until we can hold Julia and Ronan ourselves. We love you all so much!

Uncle Joe, Aunt Mary, and Kayleigh

6 July 22, 2006

Sorry we didn't post yesterday. Grandma and Grandpa went back to New Jersey this morning. Mom and Dad are now alone in the house and will need to get back into the groove of cooking and cleaning. We have appreciated everybody's efforts these past two weeks. Ronan and Julia are now two weeks and one day old. Ronan is having issues with his bilirubin, and the doctors haven't figured out why yet. The drain is still inserted in his belly, but he seems to be improving. He is a tough character who never gives up on getting better.

Julia has been opening her eyes very wide, and she is receiving treatment for her PDA. We hope the medication will do its job, and she will not have to have it surgically repaired.

7 July 23, 2006

Yesterday I noticed Julia smacking her lips. I asked if that was normal at this age, and the nurse assured me that it was. Today we heard a report that Julia was sucking on a preemie-sized pacifier. Apparently, she even had her hands up to it, and it looked like she was holding it. Sorry we missed that!

Ed didn't mention that he got his first chance to kangaroo with Julia on Friday. Dad and Julia looked very happy during their session. Hopefully, Ronan will be feeling better soon so he can get his fair share of kangaroo sessions.

Let's see what else is going on—Julia completed her first three doses of Indocin. It does not appear as though her Patent Ductus Arteriosus (PDA) has closed yet, but they are going to wait a few days and possibly give her three more doses. They can give her three courses before they have to consider other action.

Ronan is stable but remains on dopamine and hydrocortisone to regulate his blood pressure. His bilirubin levels are still high, but they have called in reinforcements from the endocrine and genetic departments to see if they have any theories on what is causing the high levels.

Ronan had a tough day as they tried to give him a new arterial line. The first attempt didn't work, so they had to try a second time. However, he had plenty of drugs and slept through most of it.

They're getting bigger!

July 23, 2006, at 10:17 AM EDT

I am so happy you started up the Web site for your twins, and I can't wait for more pictures to be posted of the little ones. We all love to see the updates and watch the progression of Julia and Ronan. Remember, the doctors said it would be a rollercoaster ride for those first few months, but that the first two weeks are critical, and now they're past that two-week mark. Yeah! Now that we're all home I'm sure we'll be stopping by to help out with whatever we can do. If you need anything, don't hesitate to call us. We'll see you (all four of you) very soon!

Amber, Gene, and Jack

Thinking of you!

July 23, 2006, at 12:05 AM EDT

We think of all four of you daily, and were glad to find out about this site so we could keep track of changes and improvements. Just want you to know that I'm praying for you, and we are so happy to hear that Julia and Ronan are such tough little fighters.

Lori, Herb, Ashley, and Jordan

8 July 24, 2006

Julia and Ronan had an uneventful day. Ronan still needs help keeping his blood pressure at an acceptable level. He has low pressure rather than high blood pressure. The doctors are still puzzled by this and will keep investigating. The surgeon looked at his drain tube and was satisfied with Ronan's progress. Ronan will be getting x-rays of his tummy and a heart ultrasound tomorrow. Today he was given a break and spent the day resting. He took a few minutes to open his eyes when Mom and Dad were talking to him.

Julia is taking a break from her PDA medicine and thus was able to take some of Mom's milk. She is doing well. Both kids have severe air leaks in their breathing tubes, but this is not currently a serious problem. Thanks again to everyone who has sent food, flowers, cookies, gifts, cards, and most importantly support. The knowledge that so many people care helps sustain us in this very difficult time.

A Big Hug for the Little Babies

July 24, 2006, at 10:33 PM EDT

Nicole and Ed:

We are thinking of you two and Julia and Ronan daily. The photos, like the babies, are miraculous. We look forward to more updates and will keep you all in our thoughts.

Keep up the kangarooing. The four of you are a great team.

Love, Amy and Evan

9 July 25, 2006

Julia and Ronan are eighteen days old today. Poor Ronan had a tough day. The surgeons decided to replace the Penrose drain to help release all the air that is trapped in his tummy. He was sedated and paralyzed during the procedure. The entire process took about fifteen minutes, and his extended stomach looked much better afterward. He was out like a light the entire time.

In case he hadn't had enough today, the eye doctor also paid him a visit. Premature infants can have issues with the blood vessels in their eyes. The eye doctor felt Ronan's eyes were developing appropriately. In fact before his minor procedure, he spent the afternoon looking at Daddy and listening to exciting stories. His head ultrasound also looked good. There is no additional bleeding. We are very happy with his reports.

Julia continues on the path toward growing stronger. She passed her brother's weight, thanks to her feedings. The doctors also said her heart murmur seems to be reduced, so hopefully her PDA is closing. Julia kangarooed with Mommy for an hour and continued with her feedings. Another day has passed, and we are very thankful for the time we can spend with our little ones. Each night we can look back on the day knowing we helped our little ones get stronger and take another step toward coming home. As hard as this has been, there is also joy in softly stroking a little head or holding a tiny hand with a finger. Just watching their eyes open and look at us as we speak softly to them is worth all the pain, worry, and anguish. We now fully appreciate the worry that all parents have for their children. Thanks again for everyone's support, and we would also like to thank UNC Hospitals. They have been incredible not only with the physical care but also the emotional side. The staff truly loves their job and the tiny lives they help save.

Take one day at a time

July 25, 2006, at 09:56 AM EDT

Nicole and Ed

Believe us—we know from experience that you have to take one day at a time, and be very patient. The babes look great—I know you can't imagine it now, but they will both continue to grow and grow, and eventually, no one will be able to tell that they were ever so small! It's very stressful, but it will be worth it in the end—Maddie was! Our love and thoughts are with you always—keep kangarooing, touching, and singing to them as much as you can! It really does the trick! (And I love that you have this site—did not know about it until today).

Love, Jen, Marc, and Maddie

Great Pictures!

July 25, 2006, at 09:01 AM EDT

Give Ronan a remote control, and he's a perfect little boy—all relaxed and having a lazy day. I'm so happy you caught little Julia with her eyes open and checking things out so we could see it too. Next you'll have to make sure you get one of her with her tiny pacifier in her mouth. They look so different than they did just a few weeks ago—different coloring and much more alert. And as soon as they start eating regularly, you'll be shocked at how much weight they'll put on! Yeah for the little ones and yeah for Mom and Dad too for keeping up all your visits and care of them. I'm sure it's hard for you, but you'll have two great little twins at home sooner than you know it! Then you'll get to experience the exhaustion and newfound addictions to caffeine like the rest of us do!

Amber

Not a bad day at all!

July 25, 2006, at 11:10 PM EDT

OK, so yeah, he had to deal with the tube again—but #1—it helped, #2—his eyes got checked, and they were OK! That is wonderful news! Yeah! As for Julia ... hmm? I'm thinking she's got a competitive streak and is just ensuring she's going to be bigger than her brother.

Hang in there, guys! I absolutely LOVE reading about them! Keep hugging, cuddling, and being with those two! They'll be home before you know it and then all the sudden they'll be two years old and saying "Mommy ... go away!"

Aimee

Week 28

10 July 26, 2006

Both kids are on ventilator support to help them breathe. Their lungs are not strong enough for them to breathe without assistance. Unfortunately, the ventilator is a double-edged sword. The oxygen that helps them breathe also damages their lungs. Only time can help their lungs grow and develop, and until then, the ventilator is their only option.

Ronan is doing much better after his procedures yesterday. His belly looks good, and he was moving around a lot and opening his eyes quite a bit. The doctors will decide in a few days if he will need surgery for his intestine. Otherwise he is stable and hopefully his tummy will heal soon so he can start eating again.

Julia (a.k.a. Ms. Piggy) is gaining weight fast; thanks to Mom's milk supply. She also had a good day but spent most of our visit snoozing. The doctors think her PDA is closing, and we are very thankful. One more day in the books. Today also marks twenty-eight weeks for them, and Friday will be three weeks since they were born. More pictures coming soon. Daddy never remembers the camera, but he will tomorrow. Thanks again for everyone's love and support. It truly means a lot to us.

So cute!

July 26, 2006, at 07:20 AM EDT

I am thrilled to see these adorable babies. At such a tender age, they already are so cute and appear to have their own little personalities. I'm sending them the vibes to keep growing and developing. Hang in there, Nicole and Ed. Those doll babies are lucky to have you.

Cousin Carol

11 July 27, 2006

It was not a good day. Today both Ronan and Julia suffered setbacks. Julia's PDA reopened, and she will need another round of medication to try and close it. The result is that a lot of fluid is leaking into her lungs. Her oxygen saturation levels are sometimes lower than they should be, and she needs more help from the ventilator to keep them at the right levels. Her treatment starts tonight, so hopefully by this time tomorrow the PDA will be closing again and hopefully for good.

Preemies often have desaturations or desats. The University of Utah tells us that a desaturation is a decrease in the percentage of oxygen found in the circulating blood supply. In premature infants, saturation below 85 percent is considered below normal. In most infants, oxygen is adjusted to keep the oxygen saturation between 92 and 96 percent.

Ronan is facing surgery tomorrow due to his NEC disease. The doctors had hoped the drain would resolve the issue, but it seems to be getting worse. Now is the time to resolve it for good. The doctors need to locate the hole and then either remove that section of the intestine or sew it closed. They are not sure exactly where it is and will need to search every inch of both the large and small intestines. There is a chance he will need a colostomy until everything heals. Although he is stable, this surgery will put a lot of strain on his body. All we can do is stay positive and let the wonderful doctors do what they need to do. We truly need everybody to send as many positive thoughts and wishes toward Ronan and Julia today. Both kids have a tough couple of days ahead of them, but we will be there to support them. On a bright note, both of the kids had their eyes open today watching Mommy, Daddy, and the nurses worry about them.

Ours prayers will be with them!

July 27, 2006, at 5:12 PM EDT

Remember, for every five steps forward, you take two steps back. They will both be in our prayers for a safe surgery, successful medication, and continued healing. You guys too . . . I can only imagine the stress and worry you are feeling. As always, if you need anything, call. When I get back in town, if there is anything I can get you, let me know.

((hugs))
Aimee

Lots of Love from NYC

July 27, 2006 at 08:45 AM EDT

Nicole and Ed: your message board is great. Thanks for keeping us so informed. It sounds like Julia and Ronan are well on their way! Please let me know if there is anything we can do. My girlfriend Daniella (the woman who had premature twins last year) offered to talk to you if you want to speak with someone who had a similar experience—a lot of the things you're dealing with Ronan and Julia sound almost identical to what her boys had. Just let me know if you would like her phone number. Her boys are almost one now and totally fine—definitely giving her a run for the money! You all sound like you're in good hands and getting excellent care. My thoughts are with you, guys!

Love, Ruth

It is amazing how there can be a whole slice of life we don't know anything about. We had no idea that miscarriages were so common, and now we are finding out that premature births are also a lot more common than we thought. Everyone knows someone who has gone through it. In fact, there are forty-five other sets of parents or so in the NICU right now going through the same thing. We are not quite ready to talk to them. We're still in a lot of shock. However, one of the mothers told the nurse to tell us that she was thinking about us. She saw how much pain we were in one day and wanted to offer her support.

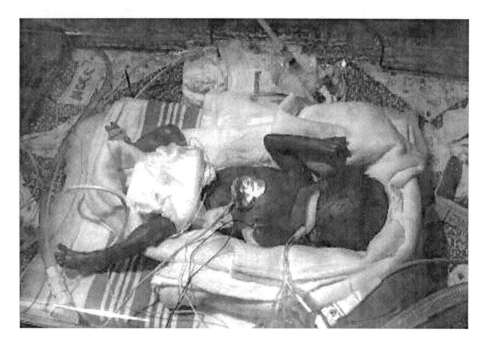

Julia, 3 days old

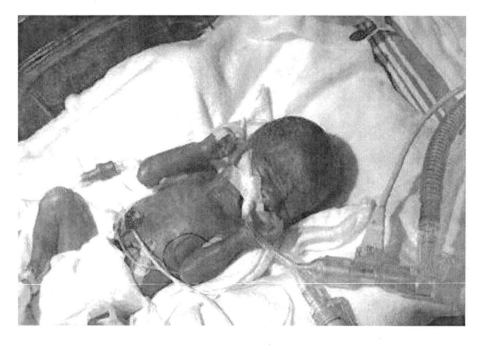

Ronan, 3 days old

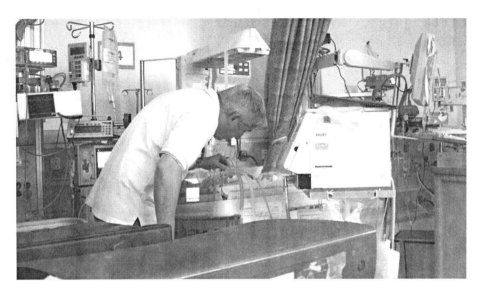

Ed with Julia in the NICU

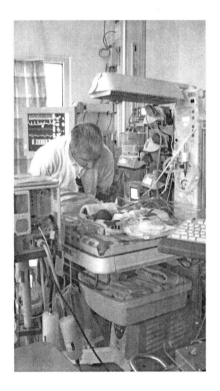

Ed with Ronan in the NICU

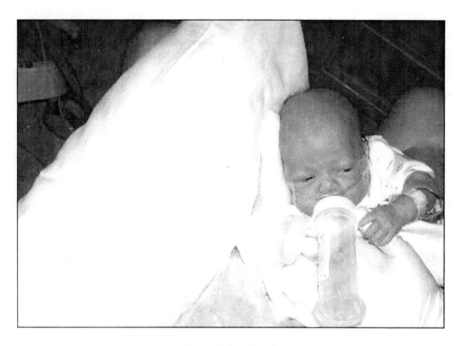

Ronan's first bottle

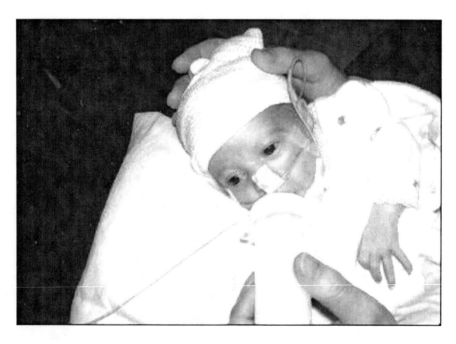

Julia's first bottle

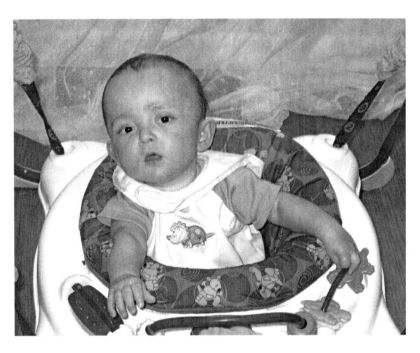

Ronan playing in his bouncy seat in June 2007

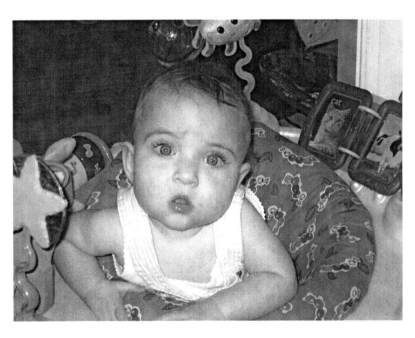

Julia playing in June 2007

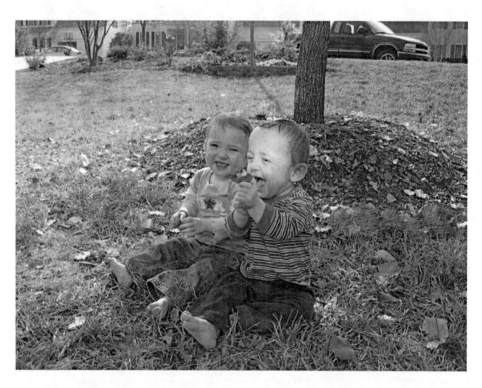

Ronan and Julia playing in the front yard in December 2007

Part 2

Riding the Rollercoaster

The rollercoaster analogy is real. Some days you'll be excited and convinced your child is getting better, and other days everything comes crashing down around you. It is important to find ways to keep your spirits up and express your feelings whether in spoken form or written form. My husband and I found that written form suited us well. We enjoyed having something to look forward to each day while at the same time keeping a record that the twins could read when they got older. It also cut down on the number of phone calls we had to return each night when we got home.

*** *How to cope*

- The NICU staff can be a vital link in surviving your ordeal. They have been through all of this with other parents and can offer you much needed support. It is amazing how much others' helping you set up and carry out an elaborate ritual around your baby's first bath, her first outfit, and her first bottle can help make the long days more bearable.
- Writing it all down—there are many sites that offer you the chance to start your own blog, and many are free.
- If you have a significant other—discuss your feelings. Don't forget that you are both hurting.

*** *How long will your baby be in the NICU?*

- There is no good answer to this. Babies do much better when they are at home. It is in everyone's best interest to get them home as soon as they are stable enough to leave the hospital.
- The rule of thumb in the NICU is that your baby will most likely be there until his original due date. Many are there for longer periods of

time, and a few are able to leave before their due date. It all depends on how they are doing medically.
  - Our daughter went home on her due date. Our son was in the NICU an additional two months after his due date.

*** *How do you handle the financial aspect of a stay in the NICU?*

- The bills for an extended stay (or a short stay) in the NICU can be staggering. Even if you have good medical coverage, co-pays and coinsurances can really add up. As a parent of a child in the NICU, you may have a social worker assigned to you. Even if you think your income might be too high, talk to your social worker about programs that might help you. If you don't have a social worker, the Internet or your local library can both be good resources for information about programs that might help you.
  - For example, because our children's birth weights were below 2 lbs 10 oz, they automatically qualified for Supplemental Security Income (SSI) during their hospital stay despite our income. In North Carolina, children who qualify for SSI automatically qualify for Medicaid. The Social Security, Benefits for Children with Disabilities pamphlet dated January 2005 states, "It can take three to five months for the state agency to decide if your child is disabled. However, we consider certain medical conditions so limiting that we expect any one of them to disable a child. In these cases, we make SSI payments right away and for up to six months while the state agency decides if your child is disabled. Following are *some* of those conditions: HIV infection, total blindness, total deafness, cerebral palsy, Down syndrome, muscular dystrophy, severe mental retardation (child age seven or older), birth weight below two pounds, ten ounces. If your child has one of the limiting conditions that is expected to disable a child, he or she will get SSI payments right away. However, the state agency may finally decide that your child's disability is not severe enough for SSI. If that happens, you will not have to pay back the SSI payments that your child got." Once they came home, we had to prove that our income was under certain limits (it wasn't), and they were dropped from the plan. However, for the time they were on the plan, Medicaid paid for the 10 percent of bills the primary insurance didn't cover. The only thing we had to pay for was 10 percent of my hospital stay and C-section. We also received SSI payments of $30 for each child each month until they were dropped from the program. You can get additional information at *www.socialsecurity.gov* or by contacting your local department of social services for more details.

- Early Intervention Program: Your child may be eligible for early intervention services if he or she shows signs of developmental delay or has high risk factors. Federal law requires all states to have early intervention programs. Call your local Children's Developmental Services Agency (CDSA) for more information. This agency provided evaluations, physical therapies, occupational therapies, and speech therapies to our children. Early intervention services vary by region.
- Community Alternatives Program for Children (CAP/C): North Carolina has a CAP/C program for medically fragile children. This is a Medicaid waiver program that is not based on the income of the parents. Programs like this vary by state. Contact your local department of social services for more details on what is available in your state. Our son qualified for CAP/C, but he is still on the waiting list.

12 July 28, 2006

Ronan went into surgery around 11:45 a.m. We spent a great morning with him. He had his eyes open for several hours and was curious about all the attention being paid to him. The surgeons think it will take a few hours to complete the operation. We are both really nervous. This is a very serious surgery, and they have no idea going in what they are going to find. I think we held our breaths the entire time he was gone. I know there was a knot in my stomach the size of a hot pretzel.

Julia has received two treatments for her PDA. Her ductis appears to be closing again. They will finish this course and hope it does the job.

13 July 28, 2006

Ronan has returned from surgery. The doctors removed several sections of his small intestine. He has four ostomy sections draining out. An ostomy is formed when a damaged piece of intestine is removed. The surgeon pulls the healthy pieces of intestine on either side of the damaged intestine up through the skin to give it time to heal before reconnection surgery. The highest ostomy will be connected to a colostomy bag to catch his waste until the intestines are reconnected in six to eight weeks.

Ronan was very stable throughout the surgery. The next few days will be critical as the intestine begins to heal and regenerate. His nutrition will be limited for several months, and he will probably spend four to five months in the hospital.

That was not quite the news we wanted to hear. Four to five additional months sounds like an eternity, and four ostomies is more than ideal. In addition, the highest ostomy is high up on his intestine, and the doctors are concerned about how much of his milk he will be able to process before it comes out into the colostomy bag.

There are two pieces of good news. One is that he has a manageable length of intestine left. It is not ideal, but they might have had to remove much more. The other is that they were able to save the ileocecal valve which is the main barrier between the small and large intestines. The ileocecal valve helps keep bacteria from the large intestine from getting into the small intestine.

The goal is to give babies a certain amount of nutrition per kilogram of weight. Most premature babies start off by receiving their nutrition through an IV. They are fed total parenteral nutrition or TPN through the IV. The National Library of Medicine Web site tells us that TPN is used for patients who cannot or should not get their nutrition through eating. TPN may include a combination of sugar and carbohydrates (for energy), proteins (for muscle strength), lipids (fat), electrolytes, and trace elements.

Long-term TPN patients sometimes suffer from electrolyte imbalances. It also can affect their liver function, causing jaundice. Providing TPN for nutrition is one of the many tradeoffs that the doctors have to make. Each time they do something to benefit the babies, there is an accompanying risk. We won't know right away whether Ronan's remaining intestine will be able to process full feeds or whether he will need to be on long-term TPN.

We are grateful that he has turned a corner and now has an opportunity to get better and grow. He still has challenges ahead, but we are finally going in the right direction. Please keep the karma coming, we will need it.

Sister Julia had a quiet afternoon, and her murmur continues to improve.

Thoughts and prayers are with the four of you

July 28, 2006, at 10:10 AM EDT

Nicole and Ed, what a wonderful journal of how the kids are doing! Nicole, I am thinking of you and sending lots of good, loving thoughts for you in this stressful time. It sounds like Miss Julia might have a touch of her mom in her! I look forward to the next update.

Ellen

Up and Down . . . and soon back up

July 28, 2006, at 09:33 AM EDT

 Of course, we're always thinking of you four here, and if you need anything at all . . . even the birds looked after, just let me know, and I'll come over. I'm just about over this stomach virus, so I hope to see you all this weekend. Can you believe the twins are three weeks old today? For being so little, they really are doing very well although I know it must not seem that way all the time. You two are doing everything right by visiting and cuddling and telling stories and such, so keep it up. I'm sure it's the highlight of the twins' day when Mom and Dad come to play.

Amber

Precious Angels

July 28, 2006, at 8:36 PM EDT

 If we never believed in miracles before, Arthur and I do now. Even though we know that it will be a while before full recovery, they are going in the right direction. The pictures are so cute that it makes us feel that we want to reach out and touch them. Julia looks very alert, and if she could talk she would probably say, "Enough already, I want to go home." Ronan looks a little out of it for now, but when he gets into shape, everyone better watch out. Arthur and I think that having twins is so cool, especially a boy and a girl. Before you know it, they'll be home in their own cozy cribs.

Love always, Roberta and Arthur

14 July 29, 2006

 Ronan has had a stable day so far today. His blood pressure medications have been pulled back dramatically and he is holding his own. The surgeons examined him this morning and were happy with his progress. He even took the time to open his eyes and say hi to Daddy. We are hoping for a quiet, stable evening and overnight. We need to take this one day at a time for the first few days.

Julia seems to be doing better today as well. She was very alert earlier this afternoon with her eyes open and tongue coming out. She even took the opportunity to poop all over Daddy when he was changing her diaper. Later, she enjoyed a ninety-minute kangaroo session with Mommy.

Overall, we had a much better day than yesterday. We are thankful for each moment that we have with our two little darlings. Peace to all and thanks again for the support.

15 July 30, 2006

Ronan and Julia passed a quiet Saturday night. Ronan has managed to stay off one of the blood pressure medications. They will slowly wean him off the other in the next few days. He was awake and alert when we came this afternoon. Nurse Dawn showed us his incision and told us that everything looks good. He is puffy and bruised, but that is all normal. An x-ray revealed normal fluid build up which should disappear in a few days. Mommy may be able to hold him tomorrow, but they won't be able to kangaroo until he heals further. Let's hope for another good day and evening.

Julia had another good night. She is still being treated for the PDA, and she will not receive any more feedings until tomorrow. She was resting comfortably when we arrived. Nurse Amy said she was busy this morning. Nurses Dawn and Amy took some time to redecorate both beds with pictures and stickers. We appreciate their helping make our little ones feel at home.

Nurse Dawn has signed up to be Ronan's primary care nurse during the day, and Nurse Katie has signed up to be Ronan's primary care nurse at night. Nurse Amy has signed up to be Julia's primary care nurse during the day, and Nurse Linda has signed up to be Julia's primary care nurse at night.

They are too high maintenance right now to have the same nurse take care of both of them. Generally the nurse gets a higher needs baby (typically on a ventilator, IV nutrition, lots of medication) and a lower needs baby (sometimes called feeders and growers) on each shift. Sometimes if the babies are feeding and growing, she may even have three babies per shift. We'll know our twins are doing better when they both have the same nurse at the same time.

On the home front, Mommy and Daddy are still working on sleep which seems to be pretty limited these days. I guess it is good practice for when the kids come home for good. Thanks for all the positive thoughts, they really help. Take care. Ed, Nicole, Ronan, and Julia.

A nice weekend

July 30, 2006, at 9:27 PM EDT

I'm glad that all of you had a fairly laid-back weekend compared to the last few weeks. It's good to have a few days with a little less stress as I'm sure there will be a few more ups and downs before they come home. But the ups will keep getting better and the downs will keep decreasing and soon this first trying month will be a distant memory. I love the newest picture of Julia. She is such a cutie, and you can already see her personality shine through! Ronan has a great personality too. He's just harder to catch on camera, I bet. Shy little boys are the best kind!
Amber

Good news!

July 30, 2006, at 12:53 PM EDT

We are so glad to hear that Ronan seems to be recovering well from surgery. The new pictures are fantastic. Love the one of Julia waving. She is looking so much like a little baby rather than a micropreemie. We'll continue to pray for their development. Can't wait to share this page with my mom when we get there. She will be amazed. Remember to take care of yourselves too!
Love, Lori

16 July 31, 2006

Ronan and Julia had another good night and morning. Julia has started her feedings again and is closing in on 1 kilogram. Ronan is not too far behind his sister. Daddy got to kangaroo with Julia today while Ronan was held by Mommy. Everybody enjoyed their time together.

Stay tuned for some pictures of Mommy and Ronan tonight. We were excited to kangaroo since Ronan hasn't been out of his bed in several weeks. Ronan's tummy looks better, and he seems to be feeling like his old self again. We are once again very thankful for a quiet, peaceful day. This is the best kind of healing possible.

17 August 1, 2006

We are closing in on one month with our little ones. Ronan is having another stable day. His intestines seem to be starting to work again, which is a big relief.

Julia is doing well also, but she will need to have a larger breathing tube inserted later today. That should help resolve the air leak which is giving her problems.

Ronan and Mommy had some more snuggle time today which is the best medicine in the world. Daddy and Julia spent an hour keeping each other warm. Nothing is better than snuggling with our babies on a lazy afternoon.

Yeah, Ronan!

August 1, 2006, at 06:13 PM EDT

I'm so happy with the progress Ronan has made these past three days. He's been such a good boy for me. I hope he continues to do well while I am off for a few days. Maybe he'll be 1 kilogram when I return! Give him kisses for me while I'm away from him!

Love, Dawn

Week 29

18 August 2, 2006

Another quiet overnight and day for Ronan and Julia. Ronan continues to be very stable. He is fighting a small infection in his stitches, but he is on antibiotics, which should help. Our little guy is a fighter and is working hard to get back in good shape.

Julia received a new breathing tube today so that pesky air leak is gone. She still has lung issues, but she needs time for them to heal and grow stronger. Her PDA is stubborn, so we'll have to go with a wait-and-see approach. Overall it was a nice, quiet, and boring day which is exactly the kind of day we like.

We would like to thank the staff at North Carolina Children's Hospital. They are the best. We really feel that our children are loved and cherished here. It is obvious this is more than a job to them. The nursing staff has been awesome, kind, and gentle with the babies and reassuring to nervous, overwhelmed new parents.

We would also like to thank everybody who has sent encouragement, prayers, thoughts, and wishes. It really makes a difference. Peace to everyone.

One day at a time!

August 02, 2006, at 04:45 PM EDT

Nicole and Ed, I am so glad things seem to be going so well for your little babes! I love reading the updates, and I am still in awe over their "toughness." I will continue to pray for their continued health as well as strength for all of you. Congratulations again, Mom and Dad . . . you have so much to be proud of!

Love,
Kathleen

Julia and Ronan

August 2, 2006, at 10:14 AM EDT

Nicole and Ed, I really can't believe it has been almost a month since your journey began. I read the message board today. It is amazing what doctors, nurses, parents, and family can do! I can only imagine what an experience this for you all. I hope the road for those sweet little ones is a smooth one from now on. Hang in there and know that my thoughts are with both daily. I love all the pictures, and it sounds like you have a great medical team on your side too. I look forward to more updates.

Barb

19 August 3, 2006

Ronan had a big day. He had a more permanent colostomy bag attached, and his breathing tube was removed this afternoon. He was a very good boy and tolerated it all very well. He is now breathing room air with the aid of a CPAP or continuous positive airway pressure mask. He spent part of the day sucking on his binky and appears to really enjoy it. His incision is still slightly infected, but the surgeon is happy with his progress. The doctors anticipate that he will begin feeding on Mom's milk on Monday. In addition, Dad got to hold Ronan for the first time today. They both seemed to enjoy it.

Julia spent some quiet time with Mom this afternoon after watching her brother get his breathing tube removed. She still has a way to go before her tube can come out. She is up to 1,042 grams and is tolerating her feedings quite well. She also is beginning to discover that she can suck, but she prefers her thumb.

Overall, a good day and we will take a few hundred more of them in a row. We have a bunch of pictures which will be posted tonight. Everybody please take care and thanks for checking in on our little ones.

Woohoo!

August 3, 2006, at 4:26 PM EDT

Jumping for joy! The people in the office are seriously wondering what I am doing! That is amazing news! Way to go, Ronan!

As for Miss Julia—she'll "catch up." Just you wait. Ed and Nicole—you might want to get back into shape now because soon, very soon, they will be running you ragged!

Way to grow, kiddos!

Aimee

Wow!

August 3, 2006, at 4:05 PM EDT

I am completely shocked (but happy) that Ronan got his breathing tube out! I wish I could have been there to witness the happy moment. I am sad that I didn't get to be present for this "big step," but I hope on Monday he'll still be doing good things without his tube! Kisses to Ronan! Hope you all have an uneventful weekend!

Love, Dawn

PS: I am so glad Julia got her bigger tube! That should make a world of difference!

20 August 4, 2006

We spent a quiet visit with the twins today. Ronan is still getting used to his new CPAP. He sometimes forgets to breathe and needs to be reminded. Of course, that makes Mommy and Daddy forget to breathe too. The biggest excitement was that Ronan was able to take some of Mommy's milk. It was just a small amount while his tummy heals, but every drop counts. He is a very good boy who always does what is asked of him.

Our friend, Rob, came to visit the kids today. They both managed to open their eyes a bit while Rob was here. Thanks for taking some time to visit, Rob!

It was great to have somebody to talk to in the pod while we visited with the kiddies. Today marks four weeks since Ronan and Julia decided it was time to come out. It's remarkable to look back at the early pictures and see how they look today. We are very thankful for having this past month with them and look forward to the future one day at a time. Monday will mark one month officially.

Ed's mother has never used a computer except for the CRT she had at work before she retired. She decided that she was going to learn so she could keep up on the progress of her "babies." One of Ed's brothers gave her his old computer and got everything set up. They showed her how to get to the CarePages. Here is her first message. She told us it took her an hour to type it.

Greetings from Stonehenge Gardens

August 4, 2006, at 10:20 PM EDT

Hi Ed and Nicole,
   This is my first message. I am so happy to see that my babies are holding their own. The new pictures are adorable. Just wanted to let you know I am thinking of you both.

Love, Mom

Great News

August 4, 2006, at 8:36 PM EDT

   Nicole, so glad to hear this good progress. Everyone on my team keeps checking on the Web site. We are all rooting for your little bundles of joy. Every day is a blessing, and the hospital is famous for their miracles. My thoughts and well wishes are with you . . . Shirley

Those darn apneas!

August 4, 2006, at 11:42 PM EDT

   I remember, in the hospital, when Emi started to turn blue. I can assure you, you'll never, ever get used to that. But as you know, Emi is two now, which means they do get over that. They won't let you leave the hospital until you have seven straight days without an apnea. Hang in there, guys! One month is an amazing and wonderful milestone! And way to go with Mommy's milk!

Aimee

21 August 5, 2006

Another quiet day for Ronan and Julia. Ronan's CPAP settings were reduced slightly, and there was even talk of his going to a nasal cannula in about a week. He also started feedings which he has been tolerating well. Daddy held him for an hour today, and he was very happy about that.

Julia is doing well too. She had a long kangaroo with Mommy. The big news is that she is up to full milk feedings, and she will no longer need a TPN supplement. They are turning off her TPN tonight. Her breathing is still an issue due to her chronic lung disease, but time will help improve that. Overall we had a very nice visit.

22 August 6, 2006

The babies had another good day. Uncle Garrett came and spent some time with them this afternoon. Ronan is looking forward to seeing Nurse Dawn. She returns from her vacation tomorrow. He was doing so well on the CPAP that they were able to lower his settings one more notch. He got to sit with Mommy for about an hour today. They both liked that a lot. They also increased the volume of his feedings, and he seems to be tolerating them well.

Julia is doing well too. They are treating her for a mild rash. She is now up to full feedings, and we're hoping she'll start to grow like a weed soon. There is a possibility that Julia could lose a little weight after she goes off TPN, but that will just be temporary.

Aww!

August 6, 2006, at 9:45 PM EDT

Thanks for the sweet note! I'm excited to see everyone tomorrow (especially Ronan of course). Tomorrow's a big day . . . one month old! We'll have to do something special to celebrate! See you soon!

Love, Dawn

23 August 7, 2006

The kiddies are one-month-old today. It has been quite a month. It doesn't seem possible that so much time has gone by, but on the other hand, it seems as if they have always been here.

Nurse Dawn had a huge surprise for us today. Somehow, she got Julia out of bed and put her in with Ronan. This is quite a feat with all of the equipment they both have on them. The pictures are absolutely wonderful. They moved Mommy to tears. The kids also celebrated by having a family picture taken together with Mommy and Daddy. Ronan is starting to become more active now that his medications have been decreased. He is feeling much better.

Julia was very squirmy today but enjoyed some snuggle time with both Mom and Dad. Mommy held Ronan briefly for the pictures. He will get some snuggle time tomorrow, for sure. We really appreciate Nurse Dawn's dedication to our miracles. Thanks again for the positive thoughts and please take a peek at the new pictures. Peace.

Good Week!

August 7, 2006, at 09:49 AM EDT

Hi Nicole and Ed, I have been on vacation for a week and just got caught on my favorite reading of the day—the twins! I am so glad they are doing so well. Lot of prayers and good thoughts are being sent your way.

Take care, Ellen

Hello from Spaghetti Night

August 7, 2006, at 7:45 PM EDT

We all just wanted to say hello the new pictures are so cute! We miss you, guys, and we're glad the twins are doing well.

Love Always,
Mina, Mary, Joe, Alana,
Bruce, Colleen, Kayleigh, and Katie

Your babies are beautiful!

August 7, 2006, at 4:17 PM EDT

Now that we get to see what they look like, they are as cute as buttons! Little Ronan is just adorable with that perfect little nose, and Julia is beautiful and has that coy smile that will just melt your heart for many years to come. Happy one-month birthday to both of them, and congratulations to both of you parents for getting to this point and doing all you do for them every day. I know you can never feel like you've done enough, but trust me, you're doing perfectly!

Amber

24 August 8, 2006

Today was another eventful day. Ronan was able to kangaroo with Mommy for the first time in several weeks. Unlike his sister, he quickly settled in and was very content. He definitely enjoys snuggle time with Mommy. Ronan is also starting to be more active. With the reduction in his medication, he is more alert and interested in his caregivers.

Julia took her first tub bath today. Mommy and Nurse Dawn slowly introduced her to the water. She was a bit nervous but managed to enjoy her first shampoo. Both kids are continuing to eat increasing amounts at each feeding which is keeping Mommy very busy. Another day of peace and quiet in Pod B. We are one day closer to coming home.

Week 30

25 August 9, 2006

Today has been a mixture of hope and fear. Ronan had his CPAP removed and replaced with a cannula (a small breathing tube inserted in the nose). He has had several episodes of bradycardia, which is very scary. The doctor recommended splitting his time between the CPAP and the cannula until he can work up to staying on cannula full time. He is a very alert little boy who likes to keep watch on Mommy, Daddy, and his favorite nurse, Dawn.

The medical team attempted to remove Julia's breathing tube. Unfortunately she did not do very well without it, and they had to reintubate her. She will be given a few days to rest and grow, and they may attempt it again next week. Her lung disease is a bit more severe than Ronan's, so she is slightly behind but will catch up eventually.

Both kids are eating well and gaining weight. Ronan is over two pounds again and is trying to catch up to his sister. Julia does not like to sleep. She is more content to look around and see what's going on in Pod B. It seems we have one calm child and one wild child.

26 August 10, 2006

Today was an uneventful day in Pod B. Ronan is back on his CPAP. The doctors decided he needs to rely on it for a while longer before trying the cannula again. His weight is good, and his feedings will hopefully go up to 4 ml tomorrow. Everything in his tummy appears to be healing well.

Julia is a wiggle worm, and she never stops moving. The nurses report she was up most of the night moving around. She seems agitated, but nobody knows for sure if something is bothering her. She does not like noise or activity near her so we have been trying to keep still and quiet around her. She needs to copy her brother and practice the art of chilling.

You've got a wiggler!

August 10, 2006, at 04:29 PM EDT

Little Julia is going to give you two a run for your money! Good thing you've got Ronan to even her out. Aww . . . but she's just a curious little thing. Hopefully when she comes home, she'll run herself ragged and then take lots of naps! Ronan will just want to hang out on the couch and watch television with his dad. Yeah for a calm day in Pod B!

Amber

27 August 11, 2006

We're having a pretty good day so far. Both Julia and Ronan gained a little weight last night. They increased the amount of calories in Julia's feedings, so Ed and I hope she'll continue to gain.

Ronan's feedings have been increased to 4 ml, and he is finally slightly above birth weight. Julia was given a sedative last night to help her to rest. She did fine on it but became super active again after it wore off. However, she did really well in her kangaroo session with Mom. She settled right in and slept like a log for the entire hour. Guess even she can't stay awake indefinitely.

Ronan snuggled with Daddy for about an hour and was very happy indeed. Both little ones continue to grow and mature. They are five weeks old today.

28 August 12, 2006

Ronan is having issues with apneas and bradycardias or As and Bs as they refer to them in the NICU. The University of Utah tells us that an apnea is a pause in breathing that may be associated with bradycardia or a slowing of the heart rate. For a premature baby less than one hundred beats per minute is usually considered a bradycardia. Premature babies have immature respiratory centers in the brain that "forget" to tell the baby to breathe. Premature infants normally have bursts of big breaths followed by periods of shallow breathing or pauses. Apnea is most common when the baby is sleeping.

Ronan is having too many As and Bs at this point, plus a build up of fluid in his body. He was given a chest x-ray, which revealed some fluid and the possibility that his lung may be collapsing. He is being treated with a diuretic for the fluid and his oxygen pressure is being increased to help his lung. There is also a chance that his darn old PDA is causing some of the problems. We'll see if the treatment improves things. Ronan got to spend an hour snuggling with Daddy. He spent most of the hour looking around and sucking on his paci.

Julia has been calmer today. She spent over an hour kangarooing with Mommy and settled down quite nicely. Her PDA is still causing her trouble, and she may have to have surgery to clip it closed once and for all. There are many different opinions on how to treat PDAs. Each doctor has his/her own theory, so we will need to see how the new attending doctor decides to handle it. All of this reinforces the fact that this is a day-to-day experience, and we should not take anything for granted. We are very, very thankful for the time we have gotten to spend with the kids. Thanks to everybody for checking in on Ronan and Julia, and please keep the good thoughts coming.

29 August 13, 2006

Ronan seems to be a bit better today. He received a blood transfusion last night and is on antibiotics again just in case there is an infection. He still has some cultures that have not come back yet. His extra fluid seems to be draining, and he was very active this afternoon.

Julia has spent a lot of time sleeping, and she is also getting a blood transfusion today. She will be monitored, and the doctors will try again later in the week to remove the breathing tube.

Glad to hear they're on the mend

August 13, 2006, at 05:29 PM EDT

We all love the adorable pictures you've been posting. It's a relief to hear those cuties are getting better again. Sounds like you're on a rollercoaster ride, down yesterday and up today. Can't imagine how hard this must be for you. But you'll all be stronger for it, so hang in there. There are a lot of people up here praying for you.

Love, Joe, Alana, and Kate

30 August 14, 2006

It was a quiet day in Pod B. Both Ronan and Julia spent a lot of time snoozing. Julia snuggled with Mommy for a while, and Ronan enjoyed his time with Daddy. Ronan continues to have As and Bs, but there do seem to be fewer of them. They are giving him more caffeine to help him with his breathing.

Julia continues the swings with her oxygen saturation levels. The doctors will attempt to remove her breathing tube later this week. Let's hope Julia decides it's time to breathe on her own. The doctors also plan on revisiting the PDA issue later this week as well.

We are very thankful for the existence of the March of Dimes. This organization helps fund research, awareness, and education for the reduction of premature births. Premature births are on the rise, and with more research funding, hospitals like UNC can help save more lives. We know that this funding has directly impacted Ronan's and Julia's chances for survival and a healthy, vibrant life. Keep thinking good thoughts for our little sweeties.

31 August 15, 2006

It was a quiet day in the pod today. Dr. Price talked to us about both kids. He is very pleased with their progress. They do continue to face challenges but are slowly progressing. Ronan continues to have As and Bs, but Dr. Price assured us they won't occur as often as he gets older. He is tolerating his feedings very well and is gaining a solid amount of weight. Ronan is also beginning to move around a lot more. He definitely feels better as evidenced by lots of wiggling.

Julia continues to wiggle as well. She is still having oxygen saturation issues, and her weight is not increasing as much as the doctors would like. She will not be able to have her breathing tube removed until she gains some weight.

The staff reminded us that patience is the key. It has already been six weeks. Some days that seems like forever ago, but on others it seems like yesterday when they arrived by surprise.

We were just told that Ronan will most likely need to go on the ventilator again. He had a couple of scary episodes today. It took quite a bit of an effort to convince him he needs to breathe. If he has one more episode, they will reinsert the breathing tube.

Week 31

32 August 16, 2006

Tomorrow is a big day. Both Nurse Dawn and Nurse Amy return from their vacations. Ronan and Julia are really looking forward to seeing them. Julia's blood gas was off this morning, and they had to adjust her ventilator, so she is going to have to wait a little longer to try extubation again. It burns so many calories to breathe that they would prefer to wait until she has gained a little more weight. She did gain some weight last night and now weighs in at 2 lbs 9 oz. If she'd stop wiggling, she could probably gain more!

Ronan weighs in at 2 lbs 10 oz although some of this is fluid weight. The staff was concerned about the severity of Ronan's As and Bs today. They took a chest x-ray to look for fluid buildup and to make sure his lungs are not collapsed. They also took an x-ray of his belly to make sure everything looked OK. They've taken some more blood to rule out infection. They increased his settings on the CPAP in hopes that they can avoid putting him back on the ventilator. That is all the news from Pod B.

33 August 17, 2006

There is not too much to report for today. Ronan received another blood transfusion. He had some nasty As and Bs during the day which really scared and upset Mommy and Daddy. He also let out some noises to let us know he has vocal cords.

Julia enjoyed an hour of kangaroo with Daddy. She is much better at it now and just snuggles in and snoozes. Ronan lost a bit of weight while Julia gained a small amount. Ronan is now up to 6 ml on his feeds, and Julia is up to 20 ml. Ronan had his fingernails clipped by Daddy, and only one tiny finger got nicked. I'm sorry, Ronan.

Mommy goes back to work tomorrow, and Daddy starts back full time. We will now see our little bundles of joy in the afternoons and early evenings.

*** *How to handle your leave of absence from work*

- As soon as you are able to, notify your manager and your human resources department of your pregnancy.
- The U.S. Department of Labor Web page summarizes the Family and Medical Leave Act (FMLA) as follows:
  - Covered employers must grant an eligible employee up to a total of twelve workweeks of unpaid leave during any twelve-month period for one or more of the following reasons:
    - For the birth and care of the newborn child of the employee
    - For placement with the employee of a son or daughter for adoption or foster care
    - To care for an immediate family member (spouse, child, or parent) with a serious health condition or
    - To take medical leave when the employee is unable to work because of a serious health condition
  - The U.S. Department of Labor Web page *http://www.dol.gov/esa/whd/fmla* defines the terms "covered employer" and "eligible employee" and gives detailed information about FMLA.
  - Your human resources department will have information about your company's parental leave and/or maternal leave of absence (LOA) policy.
- My company offered me six weeks paid LOA and six weeks unpaid LOA. I chose to return to work after six weeks so that I could save the remainder of my LOA to care for my children when they came home from the hospital. My company allowed me to take the remainder of my earned vacation time before I started the unpaid portion of my leave. I was fortunate to also be able to take an additional ninety days of unpaid personal leave before I had to return to work.
- I was pretty unhappy during the first six weeks of my LOA. The babies were both having a lot of medical problems; and the days were an unending cycle of worry, sleep, pump, worry, drive to hospital, pump, worry, visit with babies, pump, return home, worry, and start all over again.
- It was actually a relief to return to work and have something productive to occupy some of the time I previously used for worry.
- I kept in close touch with the hospital during the day and went to see the children at the NICU each night after work and on weekends.
- It was exhausting, but I found it a lot easier than being at home/hospital twenty-four hours a day, seven days a week.

34 August 18, 2006

It was a big day for Julia. She had her breathing tube removed and went on the CPAP. We actually got to see her whole face for the first time. Nurse Amy had the camera waiting so Daddy could snap some pictures for her many fans. She did pretty well on the CPAP. She still drops her oxygen saturation, but that could be caused by her PDA or lung disease also.

Ronan had a great day which included forty-five minutes of kangaroo time with Mommy. He really enjoys his time with Mommy and Daddy. His As and Bs seem to be slowing down a bit. The surgeons are pleased with how he is healing from his surgery. He was also very happy to welcome Nurse Dawn back to Pod B. Nurse Carol also stopped in to see how the twins were doing.

Woohoo for CPAP!

August 18, 2006, at 11:30 PM EDT

Woohoo! Way to grow, kiddos! You impress everyone with your steady growth and pace! Now that you don't have "masks" covering your faces, you need real pictures.

Way to go, Ronan, too! Having less A and Bs is good! They'll still be a pain in the butt, but less is more in this case!

What a great day for you, guys!

Aimee

I love these daily updates and all the beautiful pictures . . .

August 18, 2006, at 07:18 PM EDT

Hi Nicole—I've loved reading your daily updates on CarePages. Those beautiful babies—the pictures take my breath away and your daily thoughts are treasures. It will be a long road but well worth the trip! I look forward to the day I get to meet these miracles.

Mary Ellen

Good luck today!

August 18, 2006, at 09:08 AM EDT

Good luck today at work, Nicole and Ed. Just remember that you are doing what's best for your babies, and they are in tremendous hands there at UNC. Your nurses and doctors are an extension of you, but those two babies will always know who their mommy and daddy are! So work will just be a daily interruption of your baby time.

Oh . . . that's an awesome picture of your nurse holding Ronan! So nice to put a face to a name.

Aimee

35 August 20, 2006

Sorry we didn't post an update yesterday. The time seemed to get away from us. I guess we are feeling a bit overwhelmed these days. It's been forty-five days and will be at least another forty-five to sixty days, so we are wearing down a bit. We just keep focusing on keeping each other upbeat and doing whatever we can to get Ronan and Julia home.

Julia had her breathing tube reinserted this morning. She just wasn't ready for the CPAP full time. She is continuing to gain weight so we hope that in a few more days she will be off the ventilator for good.

Ronan is also growing stronger every day. He is approaching three pounds along with his sister. His As and Bs are still severe but seem to have decreased in frequency in the past day or two. One of his fistulas is leaking, but the surgeons are not concerned and continue to monitor it. We still have a long way to go before he gets reconnected. He will need lots of healing time first.

Julia is up to 22 ml per feeding, and Ronan is up to 7 ml per feeding. Both kids will continue to have their feedings increased on a slow, steady basis. Ronan gets a treat tonight as Nurse Dawn will be with him for the overnight shift.

36 August 21, 2006

Ronan had a rough night. He had a big stretch of As and Bs between 5:30 a.m. and 6:30 a.m. and nine total for the night shift. He is also having a lot of swelling of his hands, feet, and face. They will decide whether to give him more Lasiks (a diuretic) during rounds today. On the lighter side of the news, they repeated his head ultrasound, and his bleed seems to be resolving. Ronan's weight is up slightly to 1,292 grams.

Julia lost forty grams last night. She is really not gaining the amount of weight they expect, and they don't like what they saw on her x-ray today. They are considering surgery to close her PDA. They will discuss that during rounds today.

37 August 21, 2006

Julia is going to have a PDA ligation surgery this week. The doctors and surgeon agree that it's time to move forward. We are hoping it can be done as early as Wednesday, but may need to wait until Friday. The surgery involves making an incision on her left side toward the back. Once the surgeon has made the incision, she will place two clips on the offending ductis. Obviously any surgery is risky, and working so close to the aorta is also tricky. This is a very common procedure for preemies, but it still scares us to death. On a brighter note, Julia lay there bright eyed as we talked to the doctors. She even tried to turn her head over a few times.

The surgeon also checked Ronan's tummy and was pleased with his progress, but she cautioned us that problems can still occur.

Thinking of you

August 21, 2006, at 10:53 AM EDT

Hi Nicole,

Sounds like a rough night last night. Hopefully, things will be brighter today. My thoughts and lots of good energy are being sent to both of you and the beautiful babies! Thank you so much for taking the time to do the daily updates. This will be great reading for the twins when they are older.

Ellen

38 August 22, 2006

Julia is probably not going to have her surgery tomorrow. The schedule is packed, and she may need to wait for either Thursday or Friday. Today she kangarooed with Mommy and enjoyed every minute. Thanks, Nurse Amy.

Ronan snuggled with Daddy. He had a good day with very few As and Bs. Thanks, Dawn, for helping him through the day. Ronan is also up to 8 ml on his feeds, and Julia is up to 22 ml. She is getting nice and fat.

Week 32

39 August 23, 2006

We are now waiting for them to schedule Julia's surgery. The waiting is causing us a great deal of stress. She had a pretty good day yesterday, but we still worry a great deal about her. Today we found out that Ronan's and Julia's primary nurses will no longer be their primary caregivers. They will be training new nurses for a few months. They may still have the kids as an assignment but not every shift. This is a huge disappointment to us. It is very important that the nurses be very familiar with their patients. Dawn and Amy know the kids inside and out. They know what works and what doesn't work. They also know us and how we interact with the kids. They know what they can expect from us. I am going to try and talk to whoever makes these decisions. It is important that they see it from a parents' perspective. I understand the need to balance the needs for the entire department, but sometimes when doing that, it is possible to lose focus on the primary goal.

We hope to hear about the surgery schedule sometime today.

40 August 23, 2006

This news just in: Julia will have her surgery tomorrow. We don't know what time she'll have it yet, but we are hoping it will be early in the morning.

41 August 24, 2006

Julia's surgery was postponed until tomorrow. We spent a few hours in Pod B this morning since we did not find out about the canceled surgery until we got to the hospital. Julia spent that time wiggling and looking around a bit. Mommy changed her diaper, quite a challenge for a number of reasons. She gained weight last night, which is encouraging.

Ronan had a relaxing morning. He had a couple of As and Bs, but none were too bad. He had a few last night that required intervention. The neonatal nurse practitioner (NNP) told us that most of it is probably caused by immaturity. Of course, it is really scary to see one in person. The monitors start going off, the baby starts turning blue, the nurse gets out the Neopuff and "bags him" and forces air into his lungs until he is breathing on his own again.

Ronan also spent a fair amount of the visit with his eyes open. He is becoming much more active and tries to pull his CPAP mask off and wiggles himself out of his nest. The surgeon checked out his tummy and said she was going to schedule his reconnection surgery for mid-September. He still needs to get bigger and grow out of his As and Bs, but we are confident he will. She is also pleased with the amount of milk he is able to take. They are never sure how much milk a baby will be able to take after part of their intestine is removed. He passed a milestone today with his weight which is just a hair over 3 lbs. He is a bit puffy, so some of that may be fluid retention. Overall, he is looking much better these days. The kids passed thirty-two weeks gestational age yesterday, so they are still pretty young.

Tomorrow will mark seven weeks since they decided to make an early appearance. Once again we would like to thank everybody for their love and support these past weeks. It is really a big pick-me-up to read the notes. Everyone's support really helps us, especially in the hours of despair and frustration.

42 August 25, 2006

Julia went down to surgery at 7:35 a.m. Unfortunately, we were not at the hospital when she left. She originally was on the docket for the second surgery of the day, but the doctor decided to take her first. Nurse Amy reports she had a good night. She was wide-awake last night, and Amy decided to dress her up in her first outfit. It was a very pink frilly dress sewed by one of the NICU parents. When we came in, there was a very cute picture of Julia in her dress hanging by her bedside. I will scan the picture and post it tonight.

Ronan also had a good night and had his picture taken while playing peekaboo with Amy. He is on a diuretic to reduce the fluid in his system. They will also give him some acid reflux reducer today. His As and Bs may be caused by acid reflux building up in his little throat. Meanwhile he is sound asleep this morning, waiting for his sister to come back. We will post an update later today when Julia comes back from the operating room.

43 August 25, 2006

Julia is out of surgery, and everything went extremely well. The surgeon is very pleased with the results. She remained very stable throughout the procedure. She will be sedated for the rest of the day. In fact, it's the first time we have ever seen her completely still. The anesthesiologist did note that her lung disease is pretty significant, but the surgery should help her recover as she matures. Her incision is almost under her right arm and should heal quickly since kids seem to be much better at healing than adults.

Ronan also behaved himself during the surgery even though nobody was paying attention to him.

Yeah! Yippee!

August 25, 2006, at 10:50 AM EDT

Way to hold your own, Julia! Woohoo! As for the scar, you'll watch it get teeny tiny over time, and then as she grows it'll be her "freckle." Abby has two on each of her sides where the scopes went in, and they are just whiter than her normal skin. We call them her freckles.

Oh, as for the lung disease, there was a boy born at twenty-three weeks, three days who is now a thriving nearly three-year-old, and he had "significant lung disease" too, and guess what? It's 100 percent resolved! She'll heal too!

Kudos to Ronan for not doing something to get the attention back. Just wait, because when they are two, and Julia bumps her head accidentally, he'll do it on purpose to get the attention. Been there.

Aimee

44 August 26, 2006

Julia had a stable night. All her vital statistics are right where they should be. She is resting with just an occasional dose of pain medication to keep her comfortable. She was snoozing when we came in today and just briefly opened her eyes. We are still not sure when she will begin her feeds again. The doctors have not done their rounds yet.

Ronan is up to 1,442 grams or 3 lbs 3 oz. He still looks a bit puffy, but it's hard to tell which part is fluid and which part is a chubby baby developing. He seems to be reaching his limit on the volume of feeds he can handle. He was very alert when we arrived. There is even the occasional cry from him so it appears he is starting to realize he has a voice. He is still having As and Bs. The doctor's plan to check his caffeine levels tomorrow. Depending on what they find, they may increase the amount of caffeine he is being given to help decrease the numbers of As and Bs.

Precious Angels

August 26, 2006, at 06:06 AM EDT

Hi,

Let's start by asking how are Mommy and Daddy doing? Now let's continue by talking about (Tiny Classy Lady Julia) and (Tiny Mr. Macho Man Ronan). Each time I see there pictures, I want to reach out touch them and hold them. They are so adorable. It is so remarkable how much they have grown from picture to picture. It's so cute how each picture shows some expression of how they must feel with all of the equipment attached to them. The latest picture of Julia wearing a dress is so cute that it brought tears to my eyes. I think that they are starting to realize that they do not like all of the equipment on them and their expressions show it. Before you know it, they'll be home crying for their feedings and wanting all of your attention and that's worth all of the money in the world.

Love, Roberta and Arthur

45 August 27, 2006

Both kids had a good night. Julia resumed her feedings this morning since she has been doing so well after her surgery. The surgeons are very pleased with Julia's rapid recovery. There is talk in the pod that she may have her breathing tube removed as early as tomorrow. She and Ronan are both receiving blood transfusions today to give them a little boost. This should help both with their breathing. Premature babies are not ready to manufacture their own blood cells and often need transfusions. Even the relatively small amount of blood that is taken for tests affects the levels in their bodies.

Ronan is truly coming alive these past few days. He is very active and alert and reminds us he is there with a little cry every once in a while. Today, his feedings were increased by 1 ml per hour. We are very excited about that. Overall, both seem to be having a pretty good Sunday. Perhaps having Nurse Amy taking care of them today is giving them a bit of a boost.

A well deserved good-day report :-)

August 27, 2006, at 02:44 PM EDT

I'm so happy to hear the good news, and I'm positively shocked to read how well Julia is doing after her surgery! That is wonderful, and I truly hope that the surgery helped clear up the root of all her troubles so she can be back on the road to weight gain, but it will be hard to keep up with her brother—he is doing great! We know that the rollercoaster is hard on both Mom and Dad, but it's the highs like today that make the lows tolerable. Keep up all your hard work and effort for the little ones, and I'm sure they'll reward you one thousand times as they keep growing.

Amber

46 August 28, 2006

Both kids had good days. Julia is ready for full feedings and hopefully some serious weight gain followed by removal of the breathing tube. She spent our visit watching all the activity in the pod and even lifted her head up a few times to see what was going on.

Ronan kangarooed with Daddy for about an hour. He was very happy to get out of his bed. The doctors have some plans for Ronan. First, he will take Previcid for reflux. Reflux could be contributing to his A and B episodes. If that doesn't work, he may have the breathing tube reinserted temporarily so he can gain some more weight and get a bit stronger. He continues to be very alert. He was following our voices today with his eyes and was showing off how he can lift his head just like his sister. Thanks to Nurse Amy for taking care of both kids today. We know they are a handful, and we are an additional handful when we visit the pod.

Mommy and Daddy are making slow but steady progress on the nursery. Mommy is working on the dressers, and Daddy is finishing the other house projects so he can paint the nursery and put together cribs and hang pictures.

47 August 29, 2006

Both Ronan and Julia are having a good day. Mommy kangarooed with Julia who took the opportunity to snuggle in for a really nice nap. Ronan snuggled with Daddy and also took the opportunity to sleep on a warm arm. Both kids had eye exams today, and we hear that neither was thrilled with the idea. However, it is necessary to make sure their eyes are developing properly. They both got good reports. Ronan did much better on his As and Bs today; perhaps, the Previcid is working on his reflux.

Julia is up to full feedings, so we hope she will pile on the weight and make Dr. Wood happy. The kids will reach thirty-three weeks tomorrow, and the big two-month birthday is coming up next week. There is a lot to look forward to in Pod B.

Week 33

48 August 30, 2006

Ronan went back on the ventilator today. He had one too many episodes, so they decided to give him some time to rest and gain some weight. He was very appreciative and slept most of the afternoon. He did wake up enough during kangarooing to grab Mommy's necklace.

Julia slept most of the day as well. It is nice to see her save her energy toward growing and getting stronger. She woke up briefly while she snuggled with Daddy. Nurse Dawn stopped in to say hello this afternoon and reassure us Ronan is going to be fine even though he is back on the vent. Overall a quiet day that makes for a good day. The kids reached thirty-three weeks today. Boy, the days are starting to fly by.

49 August 31, 2006

Both kids had a good Thursday. Ronan kangarooed with Daddy for over an hour while Julia and Mommy snuggled. Poor Ronan lost all the hair on the front of his head. We can blame the CPAP cap for that. We are confident that the Zimmerman genes are strong in him, and he will have a shock of new hair before long. He is tolerating the increase in his feedings quite well, and his tummy is also looking good. His ventilator settings are pretty low, so hopefully a week or so of assisted breathing is all he will need.

Julia has calmed down considerably since the surgery though she still hates having her diaper changed. The doctors are slowly turning down her ventilator settings in hopes of removing her from the ventilator next week. They have also fortified her milk with extra calories so she can grow faster. It has been eight weeks since the kids decided to join us early. Some days it seems as if they have been here forever and other days it seems like July 8, a day after their birth.

Quite amazing that a baby born at only twenty-four or twenty-five weeks of gestation has a chance to live a normal life.

50 September 1, 2006

Poor Julia is having a tough day. She was agitated this morning and had some really poor breath sounds. The doctors took an x-ray and think she may have pneumonia or some more edema. She is on antibiotics and more diuretics. This is an emotional setback, but we need to realize she has pretty severe lung disease, and it will take a long, long time to resolve itself. The staff is doing what they can to treat it, but eventually time and growth resolve a lot of the symptoms.

Ronan is pretty good today. He had a nice weight gain last night, and he seems to be sleeping peacefully. He even got a sponge bath last night with a good head scrubbing. All of his remaining hair is standing on end.

Zimmerman genes

September 01, 2006, at 01:12 PM EDT

Good news! If I remember correctly, it's always a big deal to have your diaper taken away from your tush. I know I hated it . . . Also, the Zimmerman genes are good for hair? Why wasn't I notified?

Evan

51 September 2, 2006

It was a quiet day in Pod B for both Ronan and Julia though their neighbors were not too quiet. Julia's x-rays looked better today, and she seems to be peeing out the extra fluid from her lungs. She seems very content to just sleep through the afternoon. She gained about fourteen grams last night. The doctors continue to adjust her ventilator settings in hopes of weaning her down and getting her to breathe only with the assistance of the CPAP.

Ronan is doing fine as well. He is very content to sleep the afternoon away. He is now on continuous feedings to help him pack on some more weight. He is up about twelve grams from yesterday (just under 3 lbs 11 oz). Let's see if we can get him to four pounds by his second-month birthday on September 7.

52 September 3, 2006

Poor Julia is still struggling with her lung issues. I think it is going to be a long time before she has them resolved. She still managed to be wiggly yesterday and look around. She kangarooed with Daddy for a while but was not that happy about it.

Ronan is making steady progress. He is doing well on his continuous feedings. He really enjoyed his kangaroo session today with Mommy.

53 September 4, 2006

We spent a nice Labor Day afternoon with Ronan and Julia. Daddy and Ronan took the opportunity to snuggle and nap for about an hour or so. Julia and Mommy also had some snuggle/nap time. Ronan's weight was up 150 grams overnight, but it appears a lot of that was due to fluid retention. He was looking extra puffy, so he is being given diuretics to help him pass the extra fluid. It is all related to his inability to get full nutrition from milk and the need for TPN. This will hopefully compel the surgeon to reconnect him sooner rather than later this month.

Julia is still requiring a lot of energy to breathe which is keeping her weight gain to modest increases. At this point all we can do is have patience and hope she starts to gain some additional weight. She is being given fortified milk which hopefully will fatten her up a bit.

She may be struggling now . . .

September 04, 2006, at 10:45 PM EDT

But it's obvious she's a fighter. So this little battle with breathing will resolve. You are right that patience is the key. Remember that. Time heals, and these guys just need more time. I remember every day going, "When are they going to be better so they can come home?" Yes, every day I wanted that, so I know you do too. Patience and leaning on friends and family as much as possible to get you through this. You guys hang in there. I know it's tough, easy to say, tough to do. But you will get through it, just as Julia will get through these lung issues and Ronan will get through the digestive/intestinal issues.

((hugs))
Aimee

54 September 5, 2006

Ronan must be feeling left out of the worry game. He continues to build up fluid, which we can tell by the amount of weight he gained last night. The nurse today says he is extremely puffy and his lungs are sounding very "wet." They have had to increase the amount of oxygen he needs to about 40 percent. He was breathing around 21 percent which is what they call "room air" until this morning. I guess he didn't want to be left out of Mommy and Daddy's worrying.

The nurse says they are giving him additional diuretics to drain the fluid. Like everything else, the diuretics also have consequences. We were really hoping he was over these issues, and we could concentrate on getting him reattached and feeding more. I guess he has other ideas. It will be a long day at work, one filled with worry. We are planning on leaving early to go to the hospital. Once again we need everybody to keep those positive thoughts coming toward both Ronan and Julia.

Julia had an uneventful night, but her ventilator settings are still at high levels. She gained ten grams overnight.

56 September 5, 2006

Poor Ronan appears to have an infection. Dr. Wood suspects it is in his lungs. He got some blood today and is on antibiotics as a precaution. His blood gases started to improve this afternoon, and Nurse Donna says he looks much better. His feeds were stopped earlier, but they may be resumed later this evening. He really seemed like a wet noodle when we got here but had opened his eyes a few times and seems to be feeling a little bit better.

Dr. Wood also mentioned it is time to start planning his hookup surgery so that his poor liver can have a break and start getting help with positive nutrition from Mom's milk and not the nasty TPN. Improving the nutrition he receives will really help a lot of his issues. He has a lot of challenges in the next couple of days, and we are going to help him in every way we can. Also we would like to thank Dr. Wood for putting up with Dr. Sprague's Internet medicine theories. She is always willing to listen to Ed's latest readings from the always-truthful Internet.

I remember the bloating from the twenty-four weeker...

September 5, 2006, at 11:14 AM EDT

Remember the baby I keep telling you about? Born at twenty-four weeks? I remember hearing the stories about his fluid build up and the diuretics and such. He too suffered horrible lung disease. It was a battle, but I can tell you, he's a healthy nearly three-year-old with no lung disease and quite slimmed out after all that.

So, yes, worry. That's your job. But know that these are trials and tribulations that do get corrected. You guys are in awesome hands. Remember that we're all here for you too.

Aimee

Oy vey. Go raise kids!

September 05, 2006, at 05:43 PM EDT

It must seem like one step forward and two back, but I see these babies maturing in the photos as they're posted. And they are cute, cute, cute! I can well understand that you're concerned with their little insides, but hang in there. All outward signs point to maturing nicely. Hope to make it to RTP again soon so I can visit.

Love, Cousin Carol

Hey! I resemble that remark! ;)

September 5, 2006, at 06:36 PM EDT

I too had Dr. Bickers's Internet medicine theories once in the past . . . a long time ago. So I know exactly where Ed is coming from. If you have a "real" doctor who is listening, then you have found a gem!

Hang in there with the vents. Good luck with the Mommy's milk! That's some good stuff there.

Aimee

To Julia and Ronan . . .

September 5, 2006, at 05:12 PM EDT

To my favorite boy Ronan~
Be a good boy for your nurses while I am away in Vegas. I am hoping you can get rid of all your fluid and get scheduled for your surgery soon! Work on getting rid of your ventilator too. I am hoping to find you on a cannula (or at least CPAP) when I get back from my conference!
Lots of kisses!
Love, Dawn

To Julia~
Be a good girl, and start growing so you too can get rid of your ventilator soon. I want to see you and Ronan snuggled together soon!
Love, Dawn

Week 34

57 September 6, 2006

We really need everybody to think a few extra good thoughts to Ronan today. He is battling against some heavy odds, and we need all the help we can get for him. His poor little body is fighting hard, but we are not sure he has enough fight left in him. Everybody in the NICU is working very hard to help him, and Mommy and Daddy are staying all day and overnight to give him support. Please keep thinking of him and wishing him strength. His sister is helping us by behaving herself today. She too is passing on all the karma and good thoughts she can spare today.

58 September 6, 2006

Just a quick update. Ronan appears to be stable. His blood pressure has improved dramatically from this morning, and his heart rate is down. The doctors identified the infection as late onset Group B Strep, and they have him on the proper antibiotics to wipe it out. All his tests have come back improved, and his vitals are all going in the right direction. He is on a lot of different medications right now, several of which are keeping his blood pressure at a normal range. We will be staying at the hospital tonight to help him through a hopefully stable night. Thanks for all the positive thoughts today. They really seem to be working.

Julia has had a very calm day. She behaved herself for Mommy and Daddy. We think she is worried about her brother and is trying to give him the support he needs.

59 September 07, 2006

Ronan had a stable night. He was weaned off his blood pressure medications and seems to be holding his own. He was alert last evening and briefly this morning. It appears the medicines are doing their jobs, and he is feeling better.

Julia lost some weight last night but appears to be in good spirits this morning. Perhaps she is glad her brother is feeling better. Thanks to everybody for the good thoughts. They really did the trick.

Hang in there!

September 7, 2006, at 07:36 PM EDT

Boy, we can miss a lot when we don't check up on you every single day. Keep on keeping on, and we will continue our prayers for you, the kiddies, and the doctors. Ronan and Julia are both looking so perfectly chubby and adorable. Can't wait to see them at home!

Lori

61 September 8, 2006

Ronan had a good night. He gained a bit of weight, and he still looks like the marshmallow man. Nurse Betsy said he was fussy this morning during care time. She gave him a good scrubbing from head to toe. I'm sure he wasn't too thrilled about that.

Julia gained some weight overnight as well. She is starting some inhaled steroid therapy today called Flovent for her lung issues. Yesterday was the kids' two-month birthday. To celebrate Nurse Amy dressed Julia in an outfit, but she did not cooperate with picture time and then pooped all over everything. Thanks for trying, Amy, maybe next week we can get both of them together for a couple of pictures.

62 September 9, 2006

Both kids are having a quiet Saturday. Ronan is continuing to retain fluids. They cut down on his fluids to help prevent more fluid gain. Nurse Kerry showed us how to massage him to help move the fluid and increase the circulation. He seemed to enjoy having his feet rubbed, but I'm not sure about his head or chest. His blood pressure seems to be down a bit, but the nurse also thinks it could be the arterial line they are using to measure it. His cuff pressure seems to be very stable.

Julia is holding steady on her weight and has been given another dose of Flovent. She was very wiggly when we arrived, but she has calmed down a bit since then.

Keep up the good work

September 9, 2006, at 09:58 PM EDT

Hey, Ronan, I'm glad to hear you're doing better. I too like to have my feet rubbed, and maybe someday Mommy can help me when you're feeling better. Keep up the good fight. We're very proud of all four of you; you're in our thoughts every day.

Julia, glad to hear you have been feeling pretty good the last few days; you can relax now that Ronan is feeling better, you need to focus on Julia becoming stronger every day. We love you.

Please tell all of your angels (nurses) we said thanks a million.

Carol

63 September 10, 2006

We enjoyed a quiet Sunday with the kids. Mommy held Ronan, and Daddy held Julia. Ronan said it was nice to get out of his bed. It had been almost a week since he was last held. His weight is down slightly, but he is still very puffy and bloated. The doctors cut back on his feedings because he was not absorbing the entire amount. In order to compensate, they increased his fluid intake in an attempt to increase his fluid output. It seems counterintuitive to me, but he needs to have some very wet diapers in order to pass the fluid.

Julia had a nice day though she was very wiggly. She gained ten grams, so she is progressing slowly. If things go well tomorrow, they will be weaning her off the vent.

64 September 11, 2006

Ronan is having a tough time recovering from his latest illness. His blood pressure is still extremely low and this is causing him to retain fluid. He is on hydrocortisone to control his blood pressure, and he will be given another blood transfusion. We hope the combination of these two measures will increase his blood pressure and help him draw off some of the fluid. Nurse Practitioner Elizabeth thinks it could be another infection brewing, so she is double-checking all his labs to make sure they have everything covered. They've scheduled his reconnection surgery for the week of September 25. We hope that will be a real turning point for Ronan. It impresses us that through all of this Ronan still finds the strength to look around and to move his arms and legs. This little guy has been through so much in his short life. It is truly amazing how resilient he is—a true fighter. I wish I could trade places with him. He really deserves better.

Julia is also receiving another blood transfusion. She gained weight overnight. The plan is to try and remove her breathing tube tomorrow. Let's keep our fingers crossed that Julia can manage off the ventilator.

Ed and I are beginning to show signs of wearing down. Two months have come and gone with no real end in sight. While the day has some pleasures, such as seeing our little ones for a few hours, much of the day is spent trying to balance the worry, grief, and anger with the need to carry on our jobs, relationships, and the rest that life offers. We can only hope we can be as strong as our little ones. I guess we will cry a couple more buckets of tears and get a few more gray hairs before this is all over with, whenever that may be.

Oh, guys! I am so sorry!

September 11, 2006, at 09:47 PM EDT

I know there is nothing that can make it better—except for your munchkins to get better. I hurt for you just reading your thoughts today. If my three weeks were a nightmare, you must feel like you are living in a dream state that you just can't get out of. All we can do is continue to trust in the doctors, pray for you, and hope for the best. You guys are always in our thoughts and always in our prayers. Please let me know if there is anything I can do. I'm not far, and you know that.

((hugs))
Aimee

65 September 12, 2006

Ronan is continuing to retain fluid, but he seems very alert and stable. The doctors say everything seems fine, and they will just wait until his body begins to get rid of all the extra fluids. Mommy held him for a while today, and he was very happy and awake for the entire time.

Julia had a big day. The doctors removed her ventilator tube, and she is now breathing with the assistance of the CPAP. In addition, she also got to try on some of her new clothes. That was the original intention, but since she insisted on pulling her mask and feeding tube off, they dressed her and swaddled her. She has been very happy all bundled up and has maintained her body temperature like a big girl.

Nurse Dawn stopped in on her day off to pay Ronan a visit. Ronan was very pleased to see his best friend. It was sweet of Dawn to stop in to say hello. Ronan's surgery is scheduled for September 25. Next week the surgeons will run a contrast x-ray study to make a map of Ronan's insides for a guide to use when they do his hook up. Of course, Ronan will not be happy when he sees how they are going to get the contrast into his colon and small intestine. That should make his blood pressure go up. Nurse Amy also stopped in to say hi to the kids after the staff meeting. It was great to see our favorite nurses again.

He's a teenager!

September 12, 2006, at 08:14 AM EDT

Ronan must be a teenager. He's doing everything exactly opposite of what everyone tells him. When he decides that everyone else is right, then he will do it your way (and he'd better start soon, little man). We love you all, and we're thinking of you always. Please get better so that your mom and dad can stop having heart palpitations! And that Julia sure does love sleeping on her side/tummy! She is such a cutie (just like her brother)!

Amber

Week 35

66 September 13, 2006

Both kids had a good night. We never thought we'd say this, but we are happy to report that Ronan lost 140 grams last night and looks much better. He has been very active this morning.

Julia is doing well also. She gained thirty-four grams (just over an ounce) and weighs in at 1,653 grams (3 lbs 10 oz). She is doing OK on her CPAP, but her heart rate spikes when she is wiggling (which is most of the time).

67 September 13, 2006

We had a great visit. Grandma Gilda saw the little cuties for the first time since July. She was very impressed with how much they have grown. She told them wonderful stories about their future in our family. Our friend Rick also stopped by to say hello to the kids. We were happy he had some time to come out to Chapel Hill. Julia snuggled with Mommy today while Ronan snoozed. However, he woke up for about half an hour and stared at Mommy and Grandma. Nurse Dawn also came by to say hello. She will be taking care of Julia tomorrow, and Amy will have Ronan. It will be like having the whole family together again in Pod B. Julia is doing pretty well with her CPAP, so hopefully there will be no more regressing to the ventilator this time.

Ronan lost another thirteen grams during the day and looks much better. The extra fluid is not stopping him from wiggling those arms and legs. Overall a good day—we will take a few hundred more of them in a row.

Yeah for the kiddies (and Mom and Dad too)

September 13, 2006, at 10:45 PM EDT

Now make sure to tell Ronan that he is not to lose too much weight (it's a fine line, I'd guess) and tell Julia that her weight gain is great as long as it's not fluid retention like her brother's. I'll miss seeing the little Pillsbury dough boy, but we'll all be happy to have Ronan back with us instead ... so keep up the healing, Ronan, and we're pulling for you :-). Yeah for the kids (and for giving Mom and Dad a load of good news for a day)!

Amber

68 September 14, 2006

Today was a great visit. The big news was Julia was moved from the warming bed which has been her home since July 7 to an isolette which is basically an enclosed bed. She seems pretty comfortable in there. In the warming bed, she was only wearing a diaper. In the isolette, she will be able to wear clothes. They will also swaddle her in a blanket which will comfort her. In the isolette, babies practice maintaining their temperatures. In the warming bed, all that is done for them. Since the isolette is enclosed, she'll have a little more privacy. She won't be exposed to all the bustle and noise of the activity in Pod B. We think that will decrease her stress level and help her grow. She has done great on her CPAP and hasn't had any As or Bs. Grandma Gilda had the opportunity to hold Julia today for about an hour. They both seemed to enjoy it very much.

Ronan gained some weight, but the doctors have not made any changes to any of his orders. He spent the afternoon kangarooing with Mommy and really enjoyed it. He would open his eyes every so often to make sure that his mom was still holding him.

Another big event the nurses had planned was for Julia and Ronan to get together for pictures to celebrate a late two-month birthday. Julia was her usual on-the-go self while Ronan was very disinterested and kept his eyes closed. You can see the results in the photo gallery. Many thanks to Nurses Amy and Dawn for orchestrating the pictures, decorating Julia's isolette, and mostly caring so much about our children. The isolette had several great signs on it. One reads "Julia's First Condo" and another reads "Sold 9/14/06." They have really helped make these past two months bearable for us. It's amazing how these two little babies stole our hearts so quickly. With every step forward, we want to burst with excitement and pride, and with every setback, our hearts break into pieces. We would do anything to make this all go away and start their lives with peace and happiness, but we know when they come home, it will be extra special for us. This is just a test.

LOOOVE the new digs!

September 14, 2006, at 11:11 PM EDT

> Way to go, Julia! And way to go with the CPAP too! Yeah! You go, girl! Good job too, Ronan! Get those fluids out! Congrats on a great day!
>
> Aimee

Good news!

September 14, 2006, at 10:43 AM EDT

> We are so happy that things seem to be going well and that Grandma Gilda is there to support you guys and the little ones! We are thinking about you every day and are marveling at how well you seem to be holding up—the babies aren't the only strong ones in the family!
>
> Jennifer

69 September 17, 2006

We had a great weekend. Ronan and Julia enjoyed visiting with Grandma Gilda. Grandma had the chance to hold both of them. Julia is enjoying her cozy new home in the isolette. Ronan is looking much better though he is a bit on the yellow side. The extended time he has been on TPN has really taken its toll on his liver. Julia is discovering her vocal cords. When they are on the ventilator, the babies can't make any noises because the breathing tube presses on their vocal cords. She is still hoarse from the breathing tube, but she is getting louder by the day.

Ronan is scheduled to have his contrast study on Monday. This will give the surgeons a roadmap to put his insides back together next week. Not only did Ronan have a chance to snuggle with Grandma, but Nurse Dawn got to hold him for an hour on Saturday. Nurse Amy also took some time to hold Julia and get her calmed down a bit. Thanks Dawn and Amy for caring so much. There is talk Ronan will move off his ventilator in the next day or so. Julia may get a chance to try the nasal cannula tomorrow. We are hoping that we will begin to see the light at the end of this very long tunnel soon. Thanks again to everybody who has been so supportive.

70 September 18, 2006

We also had a visit on Sunday from Photographer Aimee, *http://www.pureexpressionsphotography.com/*. She took lots of pictures of Julia and Ronan and watched Julia throw a few small fits. She specializes in photographing children and babies and often does photography work in the local NICUs. Many thanks to Aimee! We can't wait to see the pictures.

71 September 18, 2006

Today was a very busy day for both kids. Ronan had his contrast study. Everything went well, and the surgeons got the information they need for his surgery. One of the surgeons, Dr. Lange, stopped by to discuss the surgery. She will reconnect Ronan's intestine and insert a line into his stomach called a gastrostomy or g-tube. A g-tube is a device that is inserted surgically through the stomach wall, directly into the stomach. The g-tube will be used to give him continuous feeds during the night or even twenty-four hours if he needs it. This will help him grow at a faster pace during this critical period where his body is growing a lot of new tissue. It is best for them to piggyback the g-tube onto an existing surgery in case he needs it, rather than having to perform a second surgery later. His surgery is scheduled for first thing Friday morning and should last several hours. Mommy and Daddy will be spending the night before he goes to get patched up. We need the good thoughts to start flowing again to Chapel Hill. Everybody did such a great job the last time, and we need some more now.

Ronan was removed from his ventilator today and was breathing on his own with the aid of the CPAP. He had a couple brief As and Bs after he was changed. His revenge for diaper changing is to stop breathing and turn tomato red with anger. Any hope for hair on his head was dashed with the dreaded CPAP cap.

Julia was switched from the CPAP to the high flow nasal cannula. It is much more comfortable than the old CPAP mask. She enjoyed a ninety-minute snuggle with Daddy. She says he has just the right spot in his arms to let her snuggle in and snooze. Her feeds were increased today, and we are hoping for some real weight gain soon. She seems to be enjoying her stay in her isolette though it's hard to see her in it. Overall, a busy but nice day in Pod B. Nurse Amy will have both kids tonight on the night shift. Nurse Dawn will take over tomorrow morning.

72 September 19, 2006

Today was a day of firsts for Ronan and Julia. We gave Ronan his first bath. He didn't seem to mind too much and appeared to snooze through a lot of it. He was getting a bit mad toward the end when Daddy was scrubbing his head. He cleans up nicely.

Julia enjoyed her first taste of milk through a bottle. She looked a bit scared and confused at first but gulped down 14 ml pretty quickly. She promptly fell soundly asleep. In terms of effort, drinking from the bottle is similar to a heavy workout for a preemie with lung issues. Thanks to Nurses Dawn and Ashley for making today so special. We left the hospital with the biggest smiles on our faces. This was probably the happiest day we have had with the twins. The little ones also received a visit from our good friend Shazia.

Ronan is getting ready for his surgery on Friday. He promises to behave and hopefully by this time next week will be recovering nicely. He will need to go back on the ventilator for the surgery but hopefully will be off it quickly. Tomorrow will mark thirty-six weeks gestational age, which leaves only one more week until they officially become full term. We are hoping to get them home in time for trick or treating. Mommy and Daddy had better finish the nursery up soon. Thanks again for all the good thoughts and messages.

We are coming closer and closer to our goal of bringing both kids home. Though we both find Chapel Hill interesting and love the staff at UNC Children's hospital, we will not miss the daily drive or the walk from the parking garage or the sounds of alarms, respirators, and suction machines. We both hear them in our sleep and can tell the desat. alarm from a temperature probe alarm to a "pump is finished and needs to flushed" alarm. I think we could both hang Ronan's TPN fluids at this point and help the doctors write orders for the day. We will not miss the ups and downs and being totally worn out at the end of each day from worry and stress.

Week 36

73 September 21, 2006

Mommy kangarooed with Ronan on Wednesday for almost two hours. He was a little grumpy due to the fact that his feedings were cut in half, but he might have enjoyed it just a little.

Daddy fed Julia with a bottle. She is still getting used to the whole idea but managed to gobble down a full ounce of milk which left only 5 ml to be fed through her feeding tube. They are going to feed her one bottle a shift until she gets more comfortable. It is a lot of work for a preemie to feed from a bottle—the challenge lies in coordinating breathing, sucking, and swallowing.

Both kids got eye exams on Wednesday. Apparently, Ronan was so angry about this that he let out some very loud big boy cries. We're getting ready for Ronan's surgery on Friday. We'll be very relieved when it is over.

74 September 21, 2006

We are at the hospital tonight staying with the kids. Ronan has been pretty agitated since about 6:30 p.m. but is finally starting to settle down. We think he is hungry since he is only getting half his feeds. He will not be any happier later since they will stop his feeds altogether in preparation for surgery.

Julia is snuggling with Mommy. Mommy tried to give her a bottle, but she was too tired. The food went into her feeding tube, and instead she stared at Mommy for a half hour.

Tomorrow will be a busy day. Once again we are asking everybody to send some positive vibes Ronan's way. We will update everybody in the morning when the big guy heads downstairs for surgery.

75 September 22, 2006

Ronan just went downstairs to surgery. He was asleep until the noisy oxygen tank woke him up. He was very alert as they prepped him for surgery. We will post another update when he comes back upstairs.

76 September 22, 2006

Ronan is back from surgery. He did very well. One of the things they worry about with this type of surgery is whether the baby will have enough intestines to process food properly. When they did the surgery to remove the damaged intestine, he had 45 cm of intestine left. This time the length had grown to 62 cm. It is very promising that his intestines grew that much in between surgeries. The surgeon said he was very "oozy" (exact surgeon term) and they had to give him a blood transfusion. His liver looked a little hard, but that was to be expected from the extended TPN use. We were also told that he will be very puffy tomorrow from fluid retention.

He was only back in his pod a few minutes when he started to open his eyes and look around. He will be on a ventilator for a few days but should be back to breathing on his own shortly. This is his turning point toward getting bigger, stronger, and healthier.

Yeah for Ronan!

September 22, 2006, at 04:03 PM EDT

Way to go, Ronan. You sure are a good little boy, and your Mom and Dad are lucky to have you. Yes, Julia, you are a good little girl too, but we could do with less flailing limbs from you. A great way to start the weekend you guys, and here's hoping Ronan is back on the road to growth and stability with some clear sailing up ahead!

Amber

77 September 23, 2006

Ronan had a good, stable night. He gained weight as they had warned, due to fluid retention. His urine output is lower than expected, and the doctors are taking steps to increase that today. He was awake this morning but is still pretty drugged up. Thanks to Nurse Lauren for all her help yesterday. I know it was a very long and busy day, but it is truly appreciated.

Julia gained forty-five grams last night and is now well over the four-pound mark. She is doing great. NNP Elizabeth said her lungs sound fantastic, and they will go down another setting on her airflow very soon. She is still getting the hang of feeding from a bottle. It is tough to remember to suck, swallow, and breathe all at the same time.

Julia!

September 23, 2006, at 10:30 AM EDT

Julia, wow four pounds! Amazing little girl. Thanks for all the hard work to get stronger. Mr. Ronan sure is getting lots of attention—but just wait until your whole family is home, and well, and I'm sure you'll be ruler of the roost! That's a beautiful picture Mom posted of you—I love to look at it and think what you'll become.

Mary Ellen

September 24, 2006

Ronan is still stable, but he gained a significant amount of fluid weight last night. The surgeons stopped by and told us that it usually takes three days post surgery for the fluid to settle in the lower extremities and start to work its way out. He was more alert today and even got a little angry during his care.

Julia is doing better with her bottle-feedings although she did lose a little weight last night. She managed to finish one whole bottle last night and one this morning. She still has her occasional fit, especially during care, but she seems more comfortable in her condo and with her nasal cannula than she did earlier this week. All in all a good start to the new year. L'shannah tovah.

L'Shannah Tovah

September 24, 2006, at 10:24 AM EDT

May the new year bring you continued strength and better and better and better health.

Evan

79 September 25, 2006

Ronan and Julia had a good day on Monday. Julia's weight is up to 4 lbs 2 oz. During our visit, Mommy gave her a bottle. She still gets quite lazy about the whole thing and needs to be reminded it's time to eat. She demonstrates with her cries that her lungs are also getting stronger.

Ronan is feeling and looking much better. He is still a bit puffy and has gained some more weight, but he is more active and alert. His incision is also looking good. His skin and eyes are still yellow, but that will go away once he begins to feed. Nurse Dawn said she heard bowel sounds in his intestine which is a good start. We hope he can start feeding by the end of this week. He has to prove he is ready by passing stool. He sat with Daddy for ninety minutes and told us it was nice to get out of bed and stretch. Hopefully, he will be weaned off his breathing tube again in the next couple of days along with several other tubes that he dislikes. We even heard that he and his sister may soon move into cribs. That will be an exciting step for them. I really think we can almost see the light at the end of this tunnel we all went into on July 7 at 5:13 p.m.

80 September 26, 2006

Julia's weight is up to 4 lbs 3.5 oz. She is still working on improving her bottle-feeding skills. She is a funny little girl. She never wants to miss anything when she is out of her isolette.

Ronan's weight was up a bit also. His catheter was removed which I am sure made him very happy. His incision is looking red, and the surgeon expressed some concern. They decided to give him some antibiotics to knock down any infection that might be brewing.

Fantastic Progress!

September 26, 2006, at 02:25 PM EDT

What wonderful progress for Ronan and Julia. I am so happy for you that they are gaining weight and growing. It sounds like Ronan is recovering nicely from his surgery, which is very good news. Take care and let's hope this is the turning point, and they are off to a wonderful new year ... still keeping everyone in my thoughts and prayers.

Ellen

Week 37

81 September 27, 2006

The twins are thirty-seven weeks today, which is considered full term for multiples. Both kids had a good night. Julia gained another thirty grams and weighs in at 1,940 grams. She almost finished an entire bottle. Good girl, Julia! Last night she took a partial bottle for Daddy but was more interested in sleeping than eating.

Ronan is doing well. His breathing tube is coming out today. They will go directly to the cannula instead of taking a detour with the dreaded CPAP mask. Nurse Dawn reported that his incision looks better today. The surgeons removed the sterostrips which will help the wounds heal. He is also starting to pass some of the fluids that have built up since his last surgery. There is a rumor that both kids may be moved to cribs in the near future. They may actually share a crib which is called cobedding.

Ronan needs a few more days of recovery and then he can start wearing clothes. Julia will wait until her brother is ready for the crib. She is enjoying her solitude in the isolette. Of course, Ronan may wonder what is happening when he is sleeping next to his wiggly sister. That girl never stops moving. Poor Ronan just likes to chill, so this should be an interesting experiment.

82 September 27, 2006

We had a good visit today. Julia did very well with her bottle. Mommy held her for almost the entire time. She spent a good deal of it watching her new neighbor who was just born at twenty-seven weeks.

Ronan was breathing with his cannula and spent ninety minutes kangarooing with Daddy. His incision is looking much better. He also learned he can move his head. He practiced this new skill while lying on Daddy. He moved his head both ways to see what was going on in the pod. He had a visit earlier in the day from his sister. They need to get reacquainted since they will be sharing quarters soon.

83 September 29, 2006

Last night Ronan kangarooed with Mommy, and Julia sat with Daddy. Ronan was repeating his trick of turning his head with his newfound freedom from the ventilator and the CPAP, but after awhile, he snuggled in and took a long nap.

Julia took her entire bottle and then settled in for a nap herself. Ronan wishes he could have a bottle too, but the surgeons haven't given the OK for him to feed yet.

84 September 29, 2006

We had another great visit with the kids. Mommy fed Julia, who is truly getting the hang of the bottle. Daddy snuggled with Ronan. He is such a big boy now that he has started to wear clothes. Nurse Dawn bought him a special outfit for the occasion. The doctors are still waiting to let him eat. He is protesting every day, but he knows what he needs to do first to prove his intestines are ready for food. Nurse Dawn said we could bring a swing in for them as they are getting big enough where they will want to enjoy some time out of their beds.

85 September 30, 2006

Ed here: Poor Ronan has an infection that apparently is resistant to some antibiotics, so he has been moved to an isolation room in Pod C. Julia also moved and is right outside the door to Ronan's private suite. Nicole and Justin are at the hospital. I am home with the stonemason. There is also a report Julia has been moved to a crib. I will update as news becomes available.

86 September 30, 2006

Nicole here: Uncle Justin arrived last night all the way from Tokyo. He certainly wins the prize for the person who traveled the farthest to see Ronan and Julia. He got a taste of the NICU rollercoaster when we arrived to find out that Ronan and Julia had been moved from Pod B because one of the cultures on Ronan's incision came back positive for Oxacillin-resistant Staphylococcus aureus (ORSA) which is easily transmittable from baby to baby. It is not uncommon for a baby who has been to surgery to pick up one of those organisms at some point. This organism is resistant to Oxycillin, and they had to isolate him so it would not spread to the rest of the unit. They had to do a lot of bed switching to get space for both kids in the same pod. Thanks to all the NICU personnel involved in this effort. Ronan has his own private isolation room within Pod C. Visitors and nurses have to put on a yellow gown and gloves in order to go in and see him. There is a lot of washing of hands involved before and after these visits.

On the lighter side of the news, Ronan finally had a bowel movement last night, and the surgeons cleared him to start taking some Pedialite. Mommy gave him his first bottle ever this morning. It contained a very small amount (6 ml) of Pedialite. He had a few As and Bs during it, but this was just his first time. I think it will take him some time to adjust to feeding with a bottle. We hope that his intestines work properly and he is able to digest his food. They will slowly work their way up on the feedings and watch him carefully for signs that there is a problem. He did seem to have more As and Bs than normal today, which concerns me. I assume they'll watch him carefully on that. He also is acting a lot more like a newborn by exercising his lungs to express his displeasure at things like his assessments.

While I was feeding Ronan his first bottle, Julia was moved to a crib. It happened really fast when I turned my back. We are a little disappointed because the original plan was to put both kids together in one crib early next week, but now that Ronan has ORSA they will likely have to be separated until they go home. Julia was really looking forward to spending some time with her brother.

Justin had the pleasure of feeding Julia her bottle today. She took most of it before she zonked out. She is getting better at the whole bottle-feeding process but has a way to go before she becomes an expert. She was also very vocal today when she wanted something. That is all the news from Pod C. Hopefully, there will be less news tomorrow.

87 October 1, 2006

Ronan and Julia had a very nice Sunday. Mommy fed Julia a bottle, and she did fantastic with it. She is really getting the hang of it. She passed the two-kilogram mark and is filling in nicely. She is a real cutie. Yesterday Julia was moved into her first crib, which means they are confident she can hold her own temperature.

Meanwhile, Ronan started to drink milk from his bottle. Daddy was able to give him one while they visited. He is still trying to get down the routine of suck, swallow, and breathe. He is a bit lonely in his isolation room, so Mommy and Daddy brought him a swing. Nurse Dawn says he is ready for a crib. He is very excited to be a big boy and get to have some fun. At least with his swing he will be able to sit and watch all the action that is going on out in Pod C. Being contagious is no fun. Uncle Justin is still visiting from Japan and has been helping feed the little ones and keeping Mommy and Daddy company. Overall, a good weekend despite our move into the isolation room.

We wonder if there is anything else they can throw at poor Ronan. Of course, everything they throw at him, he throws it back twice as hard. He is one tough cookie. And there has been some new hair growth spotted on that melon of his.

88 October 2, 2006

Ronan will no longer be lonely in his isolation since his sister has tested positive for ORSA too. We are not sure how long this will last since the doctors are talking about sending Julia home soon. She is doing really well with feedings, and her weight continues to increase. Yesterday she went down on her oxygen from 1 liter to 1/2 liter and then all the way down to .175 liters. She seems to be doing well with it. Before she leaves, she'll need a final head ultrasound to make sure there are no bleeds. Other than that, she is just about done.

She tried her swing for the first time today and really enjoyed her ride. Uncle Justin made sure to turn on the music and lights to keep her occupied. She was looking around everywhere and had to fight to keep her eyes open as she grew sleepy. She really hates to miss anything.

Ronan is still working on his feeding, and we think he will be staying for a while longer. He moved straight into a crib today and was able to bypass the isolette step because he is big enough to maintain his own temperature. We are very excited about the prospect of taking them home soon. It seemed like October would never come, but now it is here, and the really good stuff is beginning to happen.

89 October 3, 2006

Both kids had a good night. Ronan is still working on his feedings and his oxygen levels. We have been asking a lot of him this past week. We've asked him to breathe on his own, feed and maintain his body temperature. He is a very good boy, and we need to have some patience as he gets the hang of things. We have noticed his color is much better in the past few days. He is not nearly as yellow. With the increase in his feedings, the doctors can reduce the volume of his TPN which will mean less stress on his poor liver. Yesterday he had on his baseball outfit and listened as Daddy told him about the baseball playoffs. Ed said, "Ronan, you and Julia will be watching baseball games with me in April."

Julia is up to 4 lbs 10 oz. She is doing very well on all of her feedings. She enjoyed her swing yesterday, and I hope she will have another chance to use it today. She is in isolation now too, but not in the same room as Ronan. Her "isolation" consists of the curtains being drawn around her.

Mommy and Daddy are very busy working on the nursery. We should have the new wood floors in next week, followed by the furniture. We cannot wait to have our little ones home for good.

Week 38

90 **October 4, 2006**

We're feeling the full impact of the isolation. Gown on, gloves on, gown off, gloves off, repeat. It is sad that we can't touch them except through the gloves. Poor Nurse Dawn had three kids in isolation yesterday, and she went through many sets of gowns and gloves. Of course, poor Ronan is alone in his little glass box, and poor Julia is alone in her curtained isolation area. I think they miss the hustle and bustle of Pod B.

Ronan was very sleepy yesterday. He is still working hard on breathing, eating, and keeping his temperature steady. He woke up right before we left, and we put him in his new bouncy chair. Yesterday he weighed 2,500 grams or 5 lbs 8.5 oz.

Dad fed Julia last night, and she continues to do better with her feedings. She is still adjusting to the low-flow nasal cannula. She has been gaining weight steadily. Yesterday she weighed 2,085 grams or 4 lbs 10 oz.

91 **October 4, 2006**

We're doing the NICU shuffle again. One step forward, one (or more) step back. Ronan had a particularly bad spell last night. They are attributing it to reflux. They suctioned him and were able to get some secretions out. They also decided to run his feeds through his g-tube over an hour until he gets used to the volume. They will hold bottle-feedings today. They may continue to hold the bottle-feedings until they are able to decrease his oxygen settings, but that'll depend on how he is doing. He had one desat. during his feed but no other episodes during today's shift as of yet. They may do a GI study on him if this continues. He gained one hundred grams last night. We are not sure where he is putting all this weight.

Julia had a quiet night and gained seventy grams. She weighs 2,155 grams or—for those who are metrically challenged—4 lbs 12 oz.

92 **October 5, 2006**

We had a nice visit last night. Ronan is receiving his milk through his g-tube after having a nasty bradycardia early in the morning. He was fine when we got there and even woke up when Daddy was holding him. He is a very silly boy with his funny smiles and apparently has the Sprague tongue. His feeds will increase today to half of the appropriate full feed for his weight. This means they will be able to reduce the volume of his TPN. His liver has a tough time with the TPN, so this will be a big step for him.

Julia had some spit-ups after her feedings. Daddy suctioned her out, cleaned her up, and changed her outfit. This is no small feat since she has oxygen and many other lines attached to her. Plus she wiggles all over the place, and Daddy hasn't changed a little kid since the early 1990s. Julia will be moved to her own isolation room next to Ronan's. We were hoping to have her in the same room, but some obstacles prevent that from happening.

93 October 5, 2006

Julia and Ronan both had eye exams this morning. Julia's eyes looked fine, but there was one section that is incomplete in terms of growth. The eye doctor will come back in one to two weeks to make sure everything is OK. Ronan had a large fit during his eye exam. He was very vocal with his protests. One of his eyes is about the same as it was the last time. The other one did not dilate well, and the eye doctor couldn't see what she needed to see. She'll try again in one week.

Ronan had several As and Bs last night. Three required vigorous stimulation before he would come out of them, and one was self-resolving. They still think they could be caused by reflux and will continue to watch it. One option is to give him continuous feedings rather than giving them to him over an hour, but that is not an ideal solution because his tummy needs to adjust to larger feeds in order for it to stretch. The night nurse was concerned about something she saw last night (not sure what), and she ordered a septic workup. They have put him on forty-eight hours of vancomyacin (which he just came off on Tuesday) and gentomyacin just in case he does have sepsis again.

Julia was moved to an official isolation room right next door to Ronan. Things are very crowded now in the NICU, and if labor and delivery gets any busier, they may have to put the kids together in one room whether they like it or not. They'd like to have them together for growing and healing (or heeling as they say in Chapel Hill) purposes, but there are a few obstacles. One is that they can only have one monitor in there, and they both need a monitor right now. The other is that they are hesitant to put them together until Ronan starts having fewer As and Bs.

94 October 6, 2006

The kids had an OK overnight. Ronan had two spells. Nurse Linda needed to use the Neopuff once, and the other time it resolved when she removed his binky. His intestines seem to be working fine, and his kidneys seem to be working also. Right now he is receiving all his feedings via the g-tube in his stomach. The doctors want him to concentrate on breathing right now. His skin tone is looking much better. The yellow is slowly disappearing. We hope he will resolve his breathing issues soon.

Julia has gained more weight and is up to 4 lbs 15 oz. She continues to feed with the bottle but gets a bit sleepy from time to time. The big news is she is being prepared for her discharge. Mommy and Daddy will stay with her Sunday night to get used to having her around all the time. We are both very nervous and excited at the same time. Of course, we will have to leave Ronan by himself in Pod C for a while longer. This will really break our hearts, but we know he will get better. We also know that he gets lots of love and attention from Nurses Dawn and Amy and all the other great caregivers. Just writing this makes the tears start, but our big boy isn't too far behind his sister. So Mommy and Daddy have a lot of work to do this weekend to get ready. It never seemed that October would come. Now we are here, and it doesn't seem possible that we will soon have the kids at home with us.

95 October 7, 2006

We had a really great visit today with both kids. Ronan is just the sweetest baby. He looks like an angel when he is sleeping. We get a kick out of all the faces he makes when asleep. While he is awake, the eyes never stop moving. There is a lot to see, and he wants to see it all. He also loves to smile although we know he probably isn't controlling it right now. He also grunts, speaks, and squeals, which amuse us. His favorite hobby is snuggling with Mommy. He knows exactly how to get in the perfect position. His feeds have finally increased to the point where he can be removed from the dreaded TPN. His liver can now really start to regenerate and grow. His color and puffiness look much better. This week an occupational therapist (OT) is going to start working with him to loosen up his limbs because they are stiff. He will even get some water time in a small tub to stretch those arms and legs. We haven't ruled out acupuncture to get him in top form for his homecoming. Speaking of that, NNP Elizabeth thinks it could be a few more weeks, but it will depend on how well he does with his feedings and breathing. We know he will do super with Dawn, Amy, and Linda helping him out. He is also quickly outgrowing his preemie outfits and diapers.

Julia is also a showstopper. She loves to cast those dark (blue maybe) eyes upon Mom and Dad and then snuggle in deep for some quiet time. She is preparing to depart the pod for home. She is still working on her feedings. Sometimes she is a bit lazy about it and is more interested in looking around than eating. We are rooming in with her Sunday night. It should be an interesting evening.

*** *What is Rooming in and why would I want to do it?*

- Before the NICU lets you take your baby home, they may want you to room in for a night or two. You sleep in a room in the NICU with your baby overnight. You provide the care for the night, but the nurse is monitoring all the vitals and can rush in if something goes wrong.
- It is like a practice run. You get to try it all yourself in a controlled environment.
- It gave us the confidence we needed in order to do the real thing.

Rooming in! Woohoo!

October 8, 2006, at 11:31 AM EDT

Yeah, Julia! I remember that day fondly. I was scared yet excited. You will be too, I'm sure. And when you get home and start adjusting to having a baby rule every moment of your life (more than they do today, I can assure you) you'll learn all the tricks of the trade quickly!

Such awesome news! Keep up the good work, Ronan! Then you'll be home in no time!

Aimee

October 9, 2006

We had a good sleepover with Julia last night. She was a bit cranky at first, but she settled down after Daddy held her for a while. We got up to feed her at 11:00 p.m., 3:00 a.m., and 6:15 a.m. She was a bit wild at the 3:00 a.m. feeding but did pretty well for the other two. Mommy and Daddy will need some time to get used to this whole thing, but it was great to hear the little squeaks and grunts from her crib.

Ronan is doing pretty well. He still has some As and Bs, but the opinion remains that time and good feedings will make them go away. He is up to full feedings or pretty close to it, and no more TPN is hanging next to his bed. Yesterday Mommy put up a mobile for him, so he has something to keep himself busy. He also enjoys spending time in his bouncy chair and looking out the door of his isolation room. He says he will miss his sister when she goes home. However, he still has all his friends at the NICU, and Mommy and Daddy promise to come visit every day just as they have for the past three months or ninety-four days, to be exact.

97 October 9, 2006

This just in . . . Julia will not be coming home this week. The doctors are not happy with how she is breathing during feedings. She has had a couple of nasty spells today. One of them was at 3:00 a.m. with Mommy, so they want to try and work on that for the next few days. Mommy and Daddy are sad but know it will only be a few more days. Since it has already been ninety-four days, what's a couple of extra days? Perhaps we can get her room ready in the next few days. The floor people are coming tomorrow, and the oxygen company is bringing over the equipment she will need at home. We also have to get the car seat installed properly. Julia has to pass the car seat test by sitting in the car seat for thirty minutes on oxygen without having a spell. We will know more later on today when we go to the hospital.

Might be a blessing in disguise

October 9, 2006, at 06:40 PM EDT

Sad to hear that Julia has decided she isn't quite ready to leave her brother but also think it's a blessing for you as it gives you the extra time you need to finish the nursery and also less time that you will have them in two different locations. Often things happen for a reason. Keep your spirits up and give those adorable babies some extra love from our family!

Love, Lori, Herb, and kids

98 October 10, 2006

Both kids had a good night. Julia gained a small amount of weight, and Ronan lost a little. Julia had an episode with her feeding and needs some more time to get used to it. The oxygen company set up a tank in our bedroom today. It has a fifty-foot oxygen tube that reaches almost everywhere in the house. On Sunday, Sue and Ashley set up her Pack and Play while Lori scrubbed the house. We really appreciate their help. We're ready to have her home as soon as she is ready to come home.

Ronan is doing well. He was switched to a special formula that helps him more easily absorb proteins. For the science majors out there, it's a less complex string of proteins. So far he seems fine with it although we think it smells awful. The doctors observed a couple of developmental issues with him. He will be getting some help from the developmental team. They think he is slightly behind because he was sick for so long. We are all going to work with him to get him to where he belongs. He now has a bouncy seat and mobile to keep him occupied since he has to stay in the nasty old isolation room. He will have a head ultrasound when he gets closer to discharge to make sure his brain bleeds are continuing to heal.

We are also ensuring that he gets held for a while each day when we are not there. It's time to bring in the "cuddlers." Cuddlers are volunteers who take time to sit and hold the babies and give them some contact and feelings of closeness. We always chuckle at the cuddlers as they are always motivated to hold a baby. Each day they go around knocking on each pod's door asking if there are any babies that need cuddling. They are easy to spot because they all wear maroon blazers.

Week 39

99 October 11, 2006

Both kiddies had a good overnight and day. Julia lost a small amount of weight and Ronan gained some but is still looking much better. He went for an upper GI test today, and they did not see much reflux. What they did see was one angry baby who wasn't pleased with this latest test. His next test will be a scope down his throat to see if his airway is floppy.

Julia is working at her feedings and breathing. She had an A and B yesterday morning, and this will delay her coming home until next week. We will be rooming in with her on Friday night so we can feed her and learn about the signs that she is having an "episode" or, as my grandmother would say, "one of her spells." Today Julia spent a few hours swinging in her chair, and Ronan enjoyed several hours sitting in his bouncy seat. He is also beginning to enjoy the mobile we brought him. All of his favorite animals (along with musical accompaniment) spin around over his bed. A special thanks to Rich, Garrett, Lori, Sue, and Ashley who helped us get the house in order this past weekend. We are starting to see the nursery come together, and everybody was a huge help.

100 October 12, 2006

Ronan and Julia both received their dreaded eye exams today. They make a really big fuss about it. I think they are going to be scared of eye doctors for life. Julia's eyes look OK. There is one little section on each eye that is immature, but the doctor thinks her eyes will finish growing properly and doesn't want to see her again for a month. Ronan's eye exam was a little worse than last week. To be safe, the doctor will come again next week, and if everything is the same then, there is a good chance he will be fine.

Each baby has their primary nurse today, so they are very well behaved. Ronan tried extrafortified formula yesterday to help him gain weight. They also increased the volume of his feeds again yesterday. It might have been a little early for that, and they'll need to put him back to the regular number of calories for a few days. It always takes him a while to adjust to things, and they might have gone too fast too soon.

Ronan lost quite a bit of weight last night and now weighs in at 2,380 grams or 5 lbs 4 oz. Nurse Dawn is not concerned with this because she thinks he is still retaining water. Unfortunately, he did have four spells last night, but it might have been because the night nurse did not suction him. He hasn't had any today for Dawn.

Julia had a good night. She ate every three and a half to four hours and ate fifty to fifty-five grams each time. The scale said she gained one hundred grams, but Nurse Amy can't really see it on her. She'll probably go back down a little tonight.

101 October 12, 2006

We were told today that Julia will be coming home on Monday. We will stay over Friday night and part of the day on Saturday. We will believe she is coming home when we walk out the door with her. We heard more details about the eye exams. Julia's eyes are fine. Ronan, on the other hand, has a problem in his right eye. The doctor will continue to check it, but he may eventually need laser surgery to correct the problem.

Poor Ronan rarely catches any breaks, but we did learn today that his PDA closed on its own. This is one problem that will not need any surgery in the future. His feedings are going slowly. He needs time to adjust to increased amounts, and hopefully they can continue to slowly increase the volume and the calories. Children with intestinal surgery like Ronan often suffer from poor nutrition and can require TPN nutrition which we are very much opposed to because of the liver damage it causes.

Thanks again to Nurses Dawn and Amy for taking good care of our miracles. Julia will miss Amy, but she knows that her favorite nurse and best friend will come visit at home. She will also miss her brother terribly, but she will get Mommy and Daddy trained so we can handle both of them. Mommy and Daddy will probably cry a lot on Monday. It will be bittersweet, a victory of sorts, but we still must leave one behind. Someday soon, we will pull away from the hospital with our boy, and this chapter will close on our lives.

102 October 12, 2006

This is Ed. I wanted to post a separate note regarding my coworkers at Lenovo. Today during what I thought was a standard team meeting, they surprised me with a wonderful "shower." If I had my head on straight, I would have noticed everybody was dressed in pink and blue, but it went right over my head. My teammates and my good friends from my previous teams gave us extremely generous gifts and a wonderful cake. Throughout this entire ordeal, my coworkers have been incredibly supportive. Even if it was just a quick instant message, it really helped to know people were out there thinking of us.

I am also very thankful to my manager Therese and my second-line manager Sandra. They have been both supportive and understanding of my time commitments. My work hours went to almost zero for several weeks and then suffered as my mind could only focus on the little ones. I now work many strange hours, sometimes in the office, sometimes at night before bed, and when I wake up in the morning; but it's the least I can do for everybody on the team.

Thanks again, guys. We will never forget the help we received to help us get through this ordeal. And perhaps next spring after the cold and flu season, we can take Ronan and Julia to the office for a visit. I wish I could have written this better, but I guess I am just saying thank you.

What a wonderful company!

October 12, 2006, at 10:11 PM EDT

To be so supportive of one's employees is an amazing feat that so many companies just don't put stock in. Having that adult support on all fronts is such a tremendous asset. How nice of them to throw you guys a shower! Awesome!

Good luck with the Monday move to home. If you think you aren't getting any sleep now, you just wait until Monday night. Remember, if anyone offers help, take it! Don't be martyrs. All parents of twins deserve a break once in a while—in the middle of the night, middle of the day, on the weekend, etc. So take it when it's offered (read through the lines there, guys)!

Keep us posted! Keep up the good work, Ronan! Laser eye surgery is "easy" according to my uncle the ophthalmologist. Routine and simple and works wonders!

Aimee

Glad the eye exams went well

October 13, 2006, at 05:57 AM EDT

Hey guys,
I'm still out there following your daily updates and sending healing and growing vibes to my new cousins' one or twice removed . . . however that goes.

Since I know from my work that eyes can be an issue in preemies, I'm so pleased to hear that their exam results were good (with small but correctable problems at worst). Onward and upward.

Love, Cousin Carol

103 October 14, 2006

We spent our second overnight with Julia. It started off much better than the first, and Nurse Linda only had to come running into the room once. She is on demand feedings now. We wait for her to ask to eat rather than automatically giving her a bottle every three hours. They'd prefer we don't give her one in less than two hours because then she could become a "snacker" which can cause problems for the parents down the line. At this point, they don't want her to go more than four hours. Anytime between three and four hours is ideal. Nurse Linda fed her at around 8:00 p.m. while Mom and Dad got something to eat. This will probably be their last dinner out for some time. Around 9:00 p.m., we wheeled her into the sleep room and settled in with some gory videos such as *Don't Shake the Baby*. Around 10:00 p.m. we shut off the lights. Julia makes lots of noises as she sleeps. There is a lot of snorting, snuffling, and squeaking which, of course, made Mom nervous. Around midnight, she woke up, and Dad fed and changed her. All went smoothly.

At 3:30 a.m., Julia woke up, and Mom fed and changed her. Mom got nervous about a bunch of things and went to find the nurse. Her eye was puffy, she sounded congested, and she wouldn't take more than 38 ml from the bottle. Nurse Linda was very patient as she explained that sometimes they get puffy from lying in a certain position. She thought the congestion could be from irritation from the nasal cannula, and she showed Mom how to suction her. We tried with the green bulb sucker but didn't get much. She then gave it a whirl with the sucker attached to the wall and that was much more successful. Next we tried to get her to feed a little more, but she didn't want any, and we put her back to bed. Nurse Linda also reassured Mom that babies this age don't normally get colds although we need to watch out for respiratory syncytial virus or RSV. Preemies are very susceptible to RSV. At 6:30 a.m., Julia woke up again, and Linda took her back to Pod C for some blood tests. I'm ashamed to admit that Mom and Dad slept in until 9:00 a.m.

We promised Ronan that we'd still come visit him after Julia came home and that he'd get to come home someday too. He is still having As and Bs periodically. He had a bad one for Dad this morning, and NNP Kim had to pull out the Neopuff. They need to keep working on his nutrition in order to get him to grow, but it will all take time. They also have to go very slowly with him as they increase his calories and volume of feedings. He has been put on Prevacid for a few days in case his problem is reflux related. If that doesn't work, they will do a bronchostomy to find out what is going on with his airway. Most likely, though, we just need to wait for him to grow bigger and stronger for his spells to go away.

Tomorrow they will be one hundred days old. Nurse Dawn has some festivities planned in celebration of this event.

104 October 15, 2006

Ronan and Julia celebrated one hundred days of life today. Nurse Dawn brought in special cupcakes to mark the occasion. Our good friend Rob stopped by to visit the twins. He has not seen them since late July and was impressed by how much they have grown. Julia enjoyed being held by Rob.

We also had a field trip of sorts. Mommy and Daddy practiced hooking Julia up to her portable oxygen, and we went to visit Ronan. The kids snuggled for a while though Ronan refused to open his eyes for even one picture. After having Julia in his crib for a half an hour, Ronan was ready for some alone time again. Hopefully, they will not be separated for too much longer. We know he will be joining us at home soon. Nurses Dawn, Amy, and Linda, please take good care of our boy for us!

Tomorrow is the big day when we get to bring Julia home for good. We were very busy today trying to get everything in order but haven't finished yet. At least Julia will have a bed and a car seat. The rest is in progress though the nursery is very close to being finished. It will be exciting and sad, but it is the first step toward ending this story.

105 October 16, 2006

We got a call from the hospital this morning. Julia had two As and Bs last night. One was while she was sleeping and one was while she was feeding. They want to keep her a few more days until they are comfortable that she is doing better.

106 October 16, 2006

Ronan had a hydrotherapy session today. He sat in a warm bubbling tub while Nurse Dawn worked on his muscles and did stretches with him. It was reported that he enjoyed it immensely. He had a hearing test today, and his hearing is fine. He is tolerating his feedings as they work up slowly on the volumes.

Tomorrow is a big day for Ronan. He has his eye exam at noon. We're hoping that his eyes get a little better so that he doesn't have to have surgery on them. At 12:30 p.m., Pulmonary is coming to give him a bronchoscopy. The pulmonologist will examine the inside of Ronan's air passages to try to determine what is causing his episodes.

Julia had hydrotherapy of sorts also. Well, not technically, but we gave her a bath. She stiffened up like a board as she first touched the water but then relaxed a little. She was alternately crying and tolerating it. Part of the problem was that she was hungry, but we can't give her a bath after she eats. We also don't want to wake her up to give her a bath, so it is kind of tough to find a good time. She does seem to like the end when we wash her hair. We got a good look at the scar from her PDA, and it is fully healed. There is a small scar that will get fainter and fainter as she grows.

Nurse Amy had some going-home gifts for Julia. There are two very cute outfits (pink of course), socks, and a cool book about a little cricket. Daddy kind of ruined the ending before we got to read it to the kids. It's OK because I think they'll still be surprised. Many thanks to Amy!

Homeward Bound . . .

October 16, 2006, at 08:13 AM EDT

Yeah! The time has arrived for Julia to go outside for the first time and come home. Ronan won't be far behind, but just think what a service Julia is doing by breaking you two in for a baby at home! Ronan will have a breeze of a time just because Julia is doing all the hard work. You know, it's really hard to train parents—they are slow learners sometimes. We wish all of you the best, and remember, if you even have a slight problem or question, I'm only a few blocks away, so call and I'll be over in short order!

Amber

Congratulations and good luck with Julia!

October 16, 2006, at 08:55 AM EDT

It brought tears to my eyes to read the most recent post. I wish you all the best in your first few nights alone. We'll be thinking of you!

Karen

107 **October 17, 2006**

Ronan had his eye exam this morning, and his eyes are about the same as they were last time. He will not have to have eye surgery tomorrow, but they will check him again in a week. He is still waiting for his bronchoscopy.

108 **October 17, 2006**

Ronan finally had his bronchoscopy. The results were not a surprise. His upper airway is a little floppy, but his lower airway looks appropriate for his gestational age. There is nothing wrong with him that they can take any action on right now; he just needs to outgrow it. They will start his feedings again at 5:00 p.m.

Prayers do work!

October 17, 2006, at 04:52 PM EDT

Good job, Ronan! You listened to my pep talk yesterday evening. I am so proud of you! I said multiple prayers for your eyes and your bronchoscopy. And everything is exactly as I had hoped. Of course, I wish you didn't have a floppy airway, but that will improve with time. There are much worse things it could have been, so hang in there! I love you lots, and be a good boy while I am freezing in Indiana this week! Thanks to Amy for taking care of you today. I'm glad she was with you on your stressful day! Hopefully Julia will be home by the time I return to North Carolina.

Love, Dawn

Looking up

October 17, 2006, at 04:28 PM EDT

Sounds like things are looking up for you and your little munchkins. I would like to try that hydrotherapy myself. Sounds awesome! Boys always seem to need a little more time than girls. Just wait until potty training time! Still praying for you that this long ride will end sooner rather than later. Keep your spirits up.

Lori

Week 40

109 **October 18, 2006**

Today was Ronan and Julia's original estimated due date. They are officially at forty weeks. Ronan only had two episodes last night. His weight is exactly the same as yesterday, which is pretty good considering they stopped his feedings for several hours for his bronchoscopy. We hope with feedings around the clock (he is still on continuous feeds), he will gain weight tonight. He has been very alert in the mornings, and this morning was no exception. Amy put him in his swing and put it near the door of the isolation room so he could watch was going on in the pod. He seemed happy until his paci slipped out of his mouth, and he started crying. We need to get there early one morning to see him since he is always sleeping in the late afternoon/early evening.

Julia seems very alert too. Last night after her feedings, she was lying in bed looking at me intently. She gained fifty-five grams last night. She has been taking 70-75 ml every four hours. That is about 2.5 ounces! She is very close to six pounds now. Yesterday they started her on some medications for reflux, and they also turned her oxygen up slightly during feedings. She has not had an episode since Monday night. If she continues to behave herself, she may be able to come home Thursday or Friday. They tell us that babies do much better in a home atmosphere than they do in the hospital.

110 **October 18, 2006**

If Julia behaves tonight, she will be able to come home tomorrow. She has done very well this week, and it appears her episodes were related to reflux which is being treated. Mommy and Daddy are very excited to have her home and a bit nervous. We are staying calm since she was supposed to be home on Monday. She is really getting to be a big girl; she passed six pounds last night.

Ronan is also doing well. He was awake for his snuggle time with Daddy and was very alert. We are trying very hard to keep him alert and to stimulate him so he can catch up developmentally. We are concerned about his liver function which seems to still be lagging, but he is on medication to help that. We hope his increases in feedings will also help.

Congrats again!

October 18, 2006, at 10:04 PM EDT

I hope tomorrow is the big day for Julia! She has come a long way! As for Ronan, in a couple years, you guys need to read through these posts and the support responses again. Over and over you guys write about your concerns, and then the big boy shows you just how tough and strong and how much of a fighter he is! I am so amazed by his perseverance! Oh, and I just know that he's not going to let his sister top him for long. He's going to catch up and surpass "just because he can." Can't wait to see them both home, but way to go, Julia!

Good luck, Mom and Dad! Nothing will prepare you fully, but you know we're all here for you, so do ask for help!

Aimee

October 19, 2006

Ronan caused some excitement today in the NICU. Somehow his g-tube slipped out of his stomach, and he was brought down to the procedure floor where a Mic-Key button was inserted. We're not sure why they call it that, but it's smaller and easier to work with since it can be buttoned closed when not in use. Ronan had no issues with feeding after it was all done. NNP Elizabeth even hinted that down the line Ronan could be transferred to a hospital in Raleigh. That would be a much easier commute for us, but we would lose all the wonderful care we have now at UNC. We are sure Rex Hospital has a wonderful NICU, but we really love the staff and the care the kids have received at UNC. They are truly amazing people doing an amazing job. We still have time to think about it since Ronan still has a way to go before we can consider moving him.

Ronan spent some time today with the OT practicing how to use the bottle. They have a special bottle where no milk comes out so he can practice his sucking. He is also clutching his hands in the prayer position which is age appropriate behavior for newborns. It is good for developing his muscles.

112 October 19, 2006

It was a very sad and happy evening in the NICU. We packed up all of Julia's pictures and her clothes. She is leaving the only place she has ever known. We're happy to have her come home but worried that our level of care won't be up to the level she is accustomed to.

We fed Julia right before we left the NICU. NNP Elizabeth and Nurse Julie were sitting in the pod with us giving us last-minute instructions. Julia wasn't happy about taking her bottle. She was being kind of pokey and uninterested when she was drinking and then had what they call a "wet burp." Sometimes that is all they need so their tummy doesn't feel full anymore, and they'll be ready to eat more. Mommy waited a few minutes and tried again, and Julia had her first all-out projectile vomit. We're pretty sure there was almost nothing left in her tummy after she did that. It was not the best way to start her first night home, but Elizabeth and Julie did not seem phased by it. Everyone who knew Julia who was on last night came in to say good-bye. It wasn't really good-bye since we'll be back often to see Ronan.

It was so sad leaving Ronan. We know he needs to remain at the hospital to get well and grow bigger, but it seems wrong somehow to leave him all by himself. We'll still get to visit, but it will be a lot more complicated since Julia can't come to the NICU anymore because of the threat of RSV.

The ride home was uneventful. The portable alarm did not go off, and Julia slept through the whole thing. She continued to snooze as we brought her into her new home. Our birds Alexander and Zebulon were fascinated by her little squeaks and squeals. They will get used to it after everything settles down a bit, just in time for the second baby to come home. We fed her around 9:45 p.m. and put her into bed upstairs around 10:45 p.m. Right now she is sleeping. So far, so good, we'll see what the night brings us.

Part 3

Adjusting with Setbacks

112 October 20, 2006

Everyone told us the first night would be difficult, yet we all survived it somehow. Julia was very cranky and fussy from 11:00 p.m. until about 1:45 a.m. We were not able to get her to calm down. Finally we fed her and that seemed to settle her down though she did still have a somewhat restless night. Mommy fed her again around 5:45 a.m. and Daddy at 9:45 a.m. She did not do well for Daddy. She needs to learn to take all her bottles and not fall asleep. She has her first doctor's appointment today at 1:45 p.m. That is about when she should be eating, so we'll have to juggle a little. Overall, we are in good shape. We all just need to get to know each other better.

The doctor's appointment went well. Even in a pediatrician's office, people still get excited about babies. We had to strip her down to her diaper and parade her down the hall to the scales for weighing. She looks so tiny without clothes. The doctor had a full report from UNC, and she seemed happy upon examination. She patiently answered all our questions and told us to keep on doing what we are doing. She wants to see us again in a week.

Daddy volunteered today to stay with Julia so Mom could go see Ronan. It was the first day in 105 days of life that he has not seen his son. While Mom was gone, Daddy fed Julia and then she got to sit in her bouncy chair.

Ronan had a fair day. He had two fairly severe As and Bs last night and one mild one this afternoon. The volume of his feedings is up slightly, but they want to start giving him more calories to help him grow. It may take some time for him to grow out of his floppy airway and resulting As and Bs.

Tonight Grandma Gilda is coming to help out. Her help is much anticipated and appreciated.

*** *Going Home Tips*

*** *What if your child comes home with medical equipment?*

- Sometimes preemies have to go home on special medical equipment.
- It is better to have your baby home on special medical equipment than to have him remain in the NICU.
- The hospital has classes and videos to teach you how to use everything. It can be intimidating at first, but you will figure it out quickly because you will want to and you must.
  - Julia came home with an oxygen tank. They put a large oxygen tank in our bedroom with a fifty-foot extension line that reached around the house. When we went to doctors' appointments or for walks, we had a miniature oxygen tank that we carried with us. The medical equipment company provided us with all the equipment and training.
  - Ronan came home with a central line (or Broviac) and a Mic-Key button. A medical equipment company provided us with all the equipment and training.
  - Every night we hung his TPN and connected his overnight feedings.
- There were some rocky moments in the beginning and panicked calls to the medical equipment companies (all of which had someone on call at night), but we were really happy to have them at home with us, and we eventually became accustomed to handling all of their medical needs.

*** *What if you have multiples and one comes home and one has to stay at the hospital?*

- Twins (and multiples) don't always come home at the same time. This is a good thing. Although I was heartbroken that Ronan had to stay in the hospital when I brought Julia home, it was really important for us to get used to caring for one infant before we had to care for two.

** *When people volunteer to help after your baby comes home, say yes. There are many ways they can help.*

- Clean the house
- Wash and fold laundry
- Mow the lawn

- Shop for groceries
- Bring meals
- Babysit
    - If your baby needs a lot of medical attention, you may not be able to leave the house when you have a volunteer babysitter, but you can take a shower or a much-needed nap. If your baby is healthy enough, go out for an hour with your spouse. You'll be glad you did.

Welcome Home, Julia

October 20, 2006, at 11:55 AM EDT

Congratulations to the family! To Julia—I couldn't sleep last night either—sometimes that just happens (especially a first night in a new bed)! Ronan's a smartie—he's letting Sister Julia get the job of training and breaking in Mom and Dad so he won't have to deal with it all when he does get home. Sleep tight all . . . Mary Ellen

Home! And a trick for sleepy babies . . .

October 20, 2006, at 11:18 AM EDT

Congrats you guys! How exciting! And soon, soon, soon, Ronan will be on his way too!

We had sleepy eaters too. The key is that when you feed them, don't get comfortable. If you are all comfy and holding them really close, they get all warm and snuggly and sleep instead of eat.

What can you do if she starts to fall asleep?

- Tickle her feet;
- Tickle her under her chin;
- Undress her;
- Place cool wash cloths on her arms or legs;
- Change the diaper in the middle of the activity.
- Anything you can do to wake her back up. As she gets bigger, she's going to get better, but these tricks work well!
- Good luck!

Aimee

114 October 21, 2006

Mommy and Daddy were very grateful to have Grandma Gilda arrive in town last night. She immediately took charge when she arrived and started organizing things and planning. We really need the help and support. Julia was a challenge last night, but we all survived. We are still getting used to the whole situation. Her feeding schedule and volumes are a bit off track right now, but I think we will all settle into a routine. Our good friend Nurse Amy came by to say hello to Julia. She volunteered to stay while the three of us went to visit Ronan. Ronan was asleep when we got there but woke up briefly to say hello. He then enjoyed a long snuggle and snooze while Grandma held him. As usual, he woke up right at the end of our visit.

He had a good day overall. His weight is steady, and the nutritionist is going to come up with some recommendations to help him gain weight and start to push out the bad bilirubin that is keeping him yellow. The extra nutrition can also help solve his floppy airway since he will grow stronger. He was alert when he was awake and watched his mobile for a while. We think he misses his sister. Now that Julia is home, we miss him terribly. While it is exciting to have her home, there is a bit of sadness that we are not yet complete. We know this day will come and then we can really be excited, but for now, we are grateful to have both of them even though we're not together yet.

Change is hard!

October 21, 2006, at 10:53 PM EDT

I remember getting home with Joseph and feeling totally inept and not knowing what to do or how to do it and everything had just changed so much that nothing seemed right. Then, with the girls, three weeks in our NICU and I thought surely the nights at home would be easier—they were already three weeks old!

But nope! They were even harder! Every night I was in tears and the change of routine was so hard! It's amazing how a little change can disrupt your balance.

But then one day, it will all settle down and things will get back to "normal" and it will be good again! It's awesome you guys have help! That's excellent! And take heart that change is hard now, but it will get better!

((hugs))
Aimee

115 October 22, 2006

We survived a third night with Julia. It is getting a little easier, but we just don't understand why she gets so angry when we want to change her wet diaper. We are about ready to throw the machine that monitors her oxygen saturation and heart rate out the window. It goes off all the time. It goes off when it is not picking up the signal which is a good part of the time. When it is not picking up a signal, it either flashes with hyphens (-) or it gives us a crazy reading. The oxygen saturation should be between eighty-five and one hundred, and it has been down as low as seventeen several times. Fortunately we take the advice of the NICU personnel which is to look at the baby, not the monitor, but we still are frustrated with it. The representative at the oxygen company was very impressed with some of the numbers we've seen. She said Julia would not only be blue if those numbers were right, but she'd also be worse off than that. She suggested we wash the pulsox (the part that takes the readings) with water. We'll try it, but it doesn't sound like a very scientific solution.

Brave Grandma Gilda volunteered to stay with Julia while Mom and Dad went to the hospital to see Ronan. Ronan has not had any As and Bs since midnight which is an improvement over what we have been seeing. Unfortunately, his weight is not really going anywhere. The nutritionist came back with some recommendations today for a new formula that works well with babies that have GI problems; they are going to ease him onto it. It has more protein and lipids, and once he is tolerating it, they should be able to increase the calories on it too to help him gain weight. They are also going to start him on a multivitamin to help his nutrition. Growth is the only solution for his problems, and they are working hard to figure out how to help him grow.

Mommy and Daddy had a nice visit with Ronan. He was awake most of the time we were there. We each held him for a while, and he sat in his swing. While Mom was holding him, he demonstrated his amazing strength by getting a death grip on Mommy's hair and refusing to let go. That will teach her to bring a hair band with her. She has to be trained! While we were there, NNP Joanne came in to tell us that Ronan is cleared of the Orsa virus and will be moving to different digs so a new baby can be isolated in his master suite. Before we left, we put him in his adorable little Halloween outfit so he could celebrate the season. All the nurses have been wearing their Halloween scrubs, and Ronan wanted to know why he didn't get to wear any Halloween clothes.

When Daddy walked by the bonus room tonight and heard the loud hiccupping, he thought that Mommy had kidnapped Ronan from Pod C. Both kids get the hiccups a lot. Doesn't he know it runs in the family?

Those monitors are the pits!

October 22, 2006, at 08:00 PM EDT

We had monitors for a month—on both kids. The suckers would go off at 3 3:00 a.m. with no warning, with babies that didn't even move! Ugh! After four weeks, we talked our pediatrician into letting us ditch them as they were almost completely useless. The one and only time it would have been useful, it didn't even pick it up, but we did. That was the only time it would have even been useful.

So don't fret. You guys aren't alone. Those things are temperamental! Looking at the baby is always the right answer! Soon enough, you'll get a script to get rid of it!

Aimee

116 October 24, 2006

We are still trying to get Julia to sleep some more in her crib at night. This might take some more time as she is still getting used to us. There is nothing like hearing a baby cry in the middle of the night. Though we might be a bit tired during the day, we are very happy to have her home with us. She is a wonderful little girl, and we love having her all to ourselves.

Ronan had a great visit with Daddy yesterday. He was wide-awake and alert for much of the visit. He is starting to look at us more. He still will not make much eye contact, but he is focusing a bit more. He is changing to a new formula with extra calories, and we hope it will start packing on some weight. His latest liver tests show no change. We are hoping he shows some improvement next week and the yellow will eventually fade.

117 October 26, 2006

Ronan had another eye exam yesterday and it went well. The doctor said that his eye looked "slightly" improved. Perhaps this is a sign that his eyes will improve without the need for laser surgery. He has been alert and active the past few days. He really seems to be coming into his own. He will look at us now but not for very long since there is so much to see. He also turns his head and lifts it up. He started with the increased calorie formula yesterday and did well with it last night. He really needs to put on some weight because that will help his floppy airway. Speaking of his floppy airway, he has had a lot fewer As and Bs in the past week or so. Good boy, Ronan!

Julia is struggling to adjust to her new home. Feedings have not been going well these past few days. We are still struggling to get her on a regular schedule of feeding and sleeping. She is having some digestive problems so we have given her several doses of prune juice to help move things along. Apparently formula (especially the fortified kind) can slow their digestion down a lot. Nurse Amy has been by a few times to see Julia and even stayed for dinner last night. We really appreciate Amy's company and help.

Grandma Gilda has been a huge help around the house. She has been cooking up a storm, cleaning, and helping us with feedings and diaper changes. She is really enjoying spending time with her new grandchildren.

Babies have their own ideas!

October 26, 2006, at 01:38 PM EDT

Sleeping in the crib was a foreign concept to both my kids until they were at least two to three months old. Please don't stress or worry about it. She probably just wants to be with you guys more. The car seat works well as does a swing or another enclosed area—she's used to the confines of the NICU. She'll get there eventually! Call if you need some help or want company!

Love, Kara

118 October 26, 2006

Nicole here: Today I went into work to interview a contractor to help out during my leave. Much to my surprise, that was not the purpose of my visit. We entered the conference room, and there was a whole group of people holding a baby shower for me. There were even some attendees from Danbury Hall. Thanks to everyone for all the work it took to set up such a wonderful surprise and thanks for all of the amazing gifts! A special thanks to Connie who worked at least the entire weekend to create a keepsake scrapbook with excerpts and pictures from the CarePages. As the kids grow, I know we'll take it out often so we can remember how much they've changed since they entered this world.

119 October 27, 2006

Julia went to the pediatrician today for her one-week checkup. The nurse made a big deal of ferrying us through backdoors so we wouldn't have any contact with potentially sick children. When we were walking through the hall, she went up ahead and asked a father to move so we could pass. RSV is very serious in preemies, and it made us feel better that she went to extremes to make sure Julia didn't pick that up or anything else up at the doctor's office. Julia will be getting a special shot called Synagis once a month during RSV/flu season that will also help prevent her from contracting RSV (or at least lessen the severity if she does contract it). The doctor was very happy with her progress. She is up to 6 lbs 15 oz. Last week she weighed in at 6 lbs 8.5 oz. This was sort of a surprise for me because she has not been eating super well. However, she is on a higher-calorie formula and that must be one of the factors that helped.

Ronan is having a good day too. Although he did not gain weight, they upped the number of calories in his formula again, and he seems to be tolerating it well. Normal formula has twenty calories. Julia was as high as twenty-eight calories and is now at twenty-six. Ronan started at twenty calorie and went up to twenty-two calories a few days ago then to twenty-four calories today. Ronan is very happy to have Nurse Dawn caring for him today. In the morning, he did his stretches, and a cuddler held him for over an hour. He also got to sit in his swing for a few hours. When Mom and Dad got there, they helped to give him a hydrotherapy bath. He said he'd be happy to stay there all day if we'd let him. He is very alert and awake today and sucking on anything that gets near his mouth.

120 October 28, 2006

Julia, Mommy, and Grandma went for a walk on this beautiful fall afternoon. Julia enjoyed it very much. She is not eating too well today, but she did pretty well yesterday and is gaining weight.

Poor Ronan had a tough night. He had several episodes, and one needed the Neopuff. Apparently he did not sleep well overnight and has been snoozing a lot today. He lost twenty grams last night and is trying to get used to his new twenty-four-calorie formula. We're trying to be patient as it usually takes him a few days to adjust to changes in his formula.

Happy news

October 28, 2006, at 02:34 PM EDT

Glad to hear a good report from both kids today. My nephew had RSV, and it affected him for several months. It is good that they are taking precautions, despite the fact that it is another shot for her. Julia will appreciate it later, I'm sure, and so will Mommy and Daddy.

See, Julia will grow just fine even if she doesn't finish all those bottles at exactly the right time. A schedule is important for you to have your own sanity, but it will never be precisely perfect. Somehow those infants often have a mind of their own. Glad to hear they are both staying healthy!

Lori

121 October 29, 2006

It was nice again today; and Julia, Mommy, and Grandma took another walk. Julia slept through the whole thing again. She starts to get used to her new surroundings and feels more comfortable in her new home. She is certainly very comfortable letting us know when she wants something, usually her meal.

Dad stayed home with Julia while Grandma and Mommy went to the hospital to visit Ronan. We know we said last week that he was off isolation, but it's really true now. He'll be moving to his nonisolation spot in the next fifteen minutes. He had a couple of nasty As and Bs today but has been OK since Nurse Lauren deep-suctioned him and was able to get some yucky secretions out. He tolerated his new twenty-four-calorie formula so well that they increased him to twenty-six-calories. Hopefully, one of these days he'll show some weight gain to go along with the increased calories.

Grandma Gilda is going home tomorrow morning. Mommy, Daddy, Ronan, and Julia will all miss having her here. Thanks, Grandma! Your presence certainly made things easier for us all these past ten days.

122 October 30, 2006

Grandma Gilda went home this morning. Now the real fun starts. We are happy she was able to get to know her granddaughter a bit better. Now we need to get Mina Peggy down for a visit.

Mommy and Julia are spending a quiet day. It's very warm and sunny, so they took a walk down to the park and relaxed for a bit.

123 October 31, 2006

Happy Halloween! Julia is spending the evening with Daddy, handing out candy to the neighborhood kids. Ronan is spending the evening with Mommy handing out candy in the NICU. Ronan gained one hundred grams last night. The night nurse was so surprised that she weighed him three times. Some of it could be water weight. He is tolerating the twenty-six-calorie formula just fine and is up to 17 ml of milk per hour. For comparison's sake the first time he got milk this summer, he got 1 ml every three hours. We hope that the volume and calories will start translating into meat on his bones very soon. Ronan had developmental rounds today, and they are very pleased with his progress the last few weeks. They are going to add infant massage to his routine. It can help him grow. Mommy and Nurse Dawn gave him a hydrotherapy bath and did his stretches. This was his first bath lying flat in the tub, and he really seemed to enjoy it. He even opened his eyes for a few minutes. After the bath, Mommy got a lot of snuggle time with him.

Ronan has also been practicing every day with a special bottle that goes from one to five. One is sort of like a pacifier—no milk comes out. As the numbers go higher, a tiny bit of milk starts to come out. Nurse Dawn and OT Lisa want to make sure he does not forget how to suck since all his meals are going in his g-tube these days. He has been on a high oxygen flow to keep his airway open to prevent As and Bs. They are working to decrease it slowly. He got as high as 3 1/2 liters a few weeks ago and is now down to 2 1/2 liters. For comparison, Julia is at .2 liters. When they get down to 2 liters, they will give him a swallow study to make sure that he is not taking milk into his lungs. If he does well with that, he'll be able to try taking milk from a bottle again.

124 November 1, 2006

Julia went to the pediatrician today for her Synagis shot. This will help prevent her from getting RSV, a serious illness for a preemie. Ronan also got his Synagis shot today at the hospital. Julia weighed in at a hefty 7 lbs 4.5 oz. We can't believe how big she is getting. The doctor was a little concerned about her lungs. It sounds as if she may have some fluid buildup. To be safe, she sent us down for an x-ray. We hope to hear back on the results of the x-ray from the doctor later today or early tomorrow. If there is fluid buildup, they may have to put her back on a diuretic.

Ronan is OK now but had a tough morning. He had three severe As and Bs. Nurse Lauren thinks they could have been caused by his positioning in his swing. He has been fine since he went back to bed. They were going to lower him to two liters of oxygen flow today but will hold off now to make sure he doesn't have any more As and Bs. He managed to hold onto most of the one hundred grams he gained yesterday. He only lost ten of it today. Daddy is going to go see Ronan this afternoon, and Mommy will stay with Julia.

Thanks for the update on Ronan!

November 1, 2006, at 8:50 AM EST

I loved reading the update on Ronan this morning—it starts my day off with a smile. What a great kid—and what wonderful caregivers to help him out. Sounds like Julia is settling in, just hard to believe the long road she has traveled in just a few short months—and now she's handing out candy on Halloween! I wonder what Ronan and Julia will dress up as next Halloween. Thinking of you, love the posts!

Mary Ellen

125 November 3, 2006

Poor Julia is having some breathing issues. We are taking her to see the pulmonologist at UNC at noontime. She is on Lasix (a diuretic) to help decrease the fluid in her lungs. The scary part is the doctor advised us to pack a bag just in case she needs to stay overnight.

It was a very surreal ride to the hospital today. It is a very sunny fall day, and the leaves on both sides of the road have turned glorious colors, and I started thinking about this summer. Time just hasn't been moving as it should since they were born. Somehow we missed the entire summer while we worried about our little ones. I just don't understand how it can be fall already. On the other hand it seems like ages since they were born.

126 November 3, 2006

Julia is staying at the hospital tonight. The doctors are concerned about her breathing so they will observe her overnight. She is in the pediatric unit on the fifth floor right above her brother. Mommy and Daddy are exhausted and feeling a bit defeated to have Julia away from home tonight. We hope she will be coming back home tomorrow.

Ronan is still struggling to gain weight although he has been having fewer episodes. He was animated today for Nurse Amy.

When Nurse Amy read on the CarePage that Julia was going to UNC, she looked her up on the computer, managed to find us in the maze of rooms in the clinic on the first floor, and stopped down to see us during her break. She also came by to see Julia after she was assigned to her room. Thanks to Nurse Amy for stopping by and helping us get through the long day.

127 November 4, 2006

Julia had a good night. We're not sure when she will be going home. The doctors are a bit more distant in the regular pediatric unit compared to the NICU. Julia was eating this morning when we came in and seemed to be in a good mood. The nurse caring for her was very chatty, and Julia was gazing up at her and looked as though she was taking in every word. We hope to be able to bring her home tonight.

Ronan had a good night with no episodes. He has been aggravated by the nasal cannula. He seems to be developing good problem-solving skills as he works through his cannula issues. He has figured out how to turn his head and work it out of his nose and down to his chin. NNP Elizabeth and the doctor on rounds decided to go ahead and leave it out to see how he handles it. He is on room air, but they had the flow turned up to 2 ½ liters to try to keep his airway open. The nurses have been wondering if he really needs that high flow because his episodes seem to be more positional than anything. So far he has done very well without the cannula. His oxygen saturation rate has stayed very steady since he's had it out.

Without this aggravation, maybe he will gain some weight tonight. The doctors are getting concerned about his lack of weight gain. He seems a lot more peaceful since his cannula was removed, and he has had a few days to adjust to the twenty-eight-calorie formula.

The doctors are running a battery of tests just to make sure everything is normal. So far everything has been normal. One of the things they are testing him for is Cystic Fibrosis (CF). However, Nicole had a CVS test early in the pregnancy which showed fairly low odds of either of them getting CF. They are also testing his bowel movements to make sure that he is absorbing all the nutrients he needs to absorb to grow. Because his liver is compromised, it is possible he might need some sort of supplement for a while to help him absorb nutrients so he can gain weight.

Once all of the tests come back, they will analyze the results to determine if anything more can be done. If not, they may have to consider putting him back on the dreaded TPN to help him gain weight.

So here we are at day 120, pretty tired and stressed. Now we have two babies on separate floors in the hospital.

128 **November 5, 2006**

Julia is spending tonight at the hospital. One of the doctors thought he heard a murmur, so he ordered an echocardiogram to make sure everything is working fine. I talked with NNP Elizabeth, and she said all of Julia's previous echocardiograms were fine, so this is likely a fishing expedition. However, it is important to be very careful with preemies. We have seen Ronan turn from good to bad in a blink of an eye, and we understand the need now to be overly cautious.

Julia seemed to be in very good spirits this afternoon. Nurse Amy said she would stop by after her shift to say hello. It was hard leaving her tonight. Julia was lying in that oversized crib watching us as we said good-bye. The house is too quiet now. It doesn't take too long to get used to her being home. She should return home sometime tomorrow.

129 **November 5, 2006**

The kids are one hundred twenty-one days old today.

The pediatric unit is not as forthcoming with information as the NICU. When I talk to the nurses, they give me only limited information. I'm spoiled from getting the detailed reports I usually receive from the NICU. I spoke to them about 9:00 a.m., and they didn't have a lot to tell me. They did report that Julia tested negative for RSV. However, at 11:00 a.m. they called to say that they wanted to discharge her. We're very happy that she'll be able to come home today.

Nurse Dawn is caring for Ronan today. She bought him an adorable striped outfit with lots of animals on it. He looks very cute in it. He seems to be doing very well without his cannula. He did not have any episodes last night although he did have one this morning. Nurse Dawn is very happy with his behavior.

He is acting more like a full-term newborn. He holds his hands in front of him as he should and makes eye contact. He has also been aware of his surroundings and is having longer periods where he is awake. Unfortunately, he did not gain any weight last night. He still weighs 2,500 grams which is 5 1/2 pounds. We had a long talk with him this afternoon and told him that he really needs to gain weight so he can come home and be with his sister again. Nurse Dawn promises to visit even if he goes home.

130 November 6, 2006

Julia is finally at home and now it is Ronan's turn to worry us. One of his labs showed his sodium levels are very high. Another lab reported a urinary tract infection and dehydration. Information about how he is actually doing today was not really available since once again he has a new nurse who has never cared for him. She passed us off to the NNP Rani who provided the update. They are doing some more testing and will have additional information after rounds this morning.

Sometimes it seems that Ronan will never catch a break. He is alert and attentive these days and is making great strides with his development. He just needs his body to give him a chance to be a normal, healthy baby. Apparently stress knows no boundaries. After worrying about Julia being in the hospital with only minimal attention and being exposed to every germ known to mankind, we now have to deal with poor Ronan. At what point will it be decided that Ed and Nicole have had enough? We would gladly suffer more if it resulted in Ronan being healthy and ready to come home. Let's hope the staff has some new and more conclusive ideas of what is going on and how to treat it and get him home.

131 November 6, 2006

Ronan has to go back on partial TPN feedings. He is not absorbing enough fats and proteins to grow properly. Of course this means that his liver will be under assault from the TPN again. Sometimes the cure is as bad as the disease. His direct bilirubin readings have risen again, and he will need an ultrasound to see if there is a blockage in his bile duct. We are beside ourselves with grief and frustration because there is nothing we can do to help him. At some point we will be unable to take any more of this, and I think that point is coming very soon. The stress of taking care of one infant who has her own challenges while running back and forth to the hospital to visit another who is very sick is very difficult.

I'm so sorry

November 6, 2006, at 04:07 PM EST

You just really don't get a break, do you? I will pray that things stabilize soon.

Karen

Hang in there! If any family can do it—it's yours!

November 6, 2006, at 04:00 PM EST

We all know the stress is so hard but hang in there! You've come so far and cannot give up now! Keep fighting, Ronan! We're praying for each and every one of you every day!

Mary Lou

Hang in there!

November 6, 2006, at 07:59 PM EST

It's amazing how many times, we as parents get to the breaking point and then something good happens that keeps us moving again. You will find that strength. You are parents, and somehow, we always do.
Hang in there! Prayers for Ronan that this is just a minor setback!

((hugs))
Aimee

Heads up!

November 6, 2006, at 04:34 PM EST

I so wish there was more your friends could do to help rather than just reading your news every day. We are all out here thinking of you and wishing we could help bear the load. Know that prayer can move mountains! Stay strong!

Lori

132 **November 7, 2006**

We had a long talk with the doctor last night about Ronan. She is running a series of test to find out exactly why he is having trouble absorbing fats and proteins. It could be his liver, pancreas, or intestines. In the short-term, the TPN will help him gain weight and grow. The majority of his nutrition will still be provided by formula, and he will only receive 25 percent of his nutrition by TPN. We hope this will not damage his liver any further.

She made us feel much better though she did dash our hopes of having him home by Thanksgiving. Maybe he'll be home by Mommy's birthday on December 10. Today is the twins' four-month birthday. Julia is spending it with Mommy. Ronan is spending it with his best buddy, Nurse Dawn. Mom will go see him tonight. We hope our friend Amy will also be in Pod C today. A big thanks to Amy for watching Julia last night. It meant so much to have the chance for Ed and me to talk to the doctor.

133 November 7, 2006

They had to stop Ronan's feedings for a few hours in order to give him an ultrasound, but he took it like a trouper. The official report is not yet in; but unofficially his liver, kidneys, and pancreas all look acceptable. The plan is to consult with the gastrointestinal doctors about the malabsorption of fats in his GI tract. They will also keep him on partial TPN feedings for five to seven days. Although we are nervous about the TPN causing more damage to the liver, it is important that he receive some nutrients so he can resume growing. We're hoping that a small amount of TPN over a short period of time will not harm his liver further. Ronan is on antibiotics for his urinary tract infection. The high sodium levels and the dehydration are puzzling everyone. However, after giving him IV fluids yesterday to rehydrate him, his sodium levels are closer to normal.

Julia had a rather quiet day. She didn't get to take a walk because of the pouring rain. She is eating well, but her tendency to spit up is concerning to us. We've tried holding her upright for ten to fifteen minutes after each feed to decrease the chance of spit-ups, but it does not seem to help much. Sometimes the milk comes out of her mouth and nose, and sometimes it can cause an A and B. The weird thing is that sometimes she doesn't spit up for a good hour after she's eaten. I have a call into the pediatrician to see if she has any ideas for us.

In July, the NICU gave us a journal for each child. It has places to record their vital statistics and their milestones. I've finally started to work on it. It is very hard to remember the details of what happened in the beginning although the scrapbook Connie created helps if we mentioned the milestone in the CarePages. I've enjoyed going through my picture stash to find appropriate pictures for each page. Day to day we forget how far they've come.

Strong Will

November 7, 2006, at 04:05 PM EST

Blessing and peace. I'm so glad you have an action plan and a holiday season to look forward to as a full family. Ronan will grow big and strong—he's having a rough go at the moment, but finding the right treatment plan is half the battle . . . and you know that plan may change too as his body changes. Keep up the love and persistence to get him through this; he needs you!

Mary Ellen

November 8, 2006

Julia's pediatrician called back today and suggested I bring her into the office this morning. Luckily, she attended a timely lecture this morning about reflux presented by a neonatologist from UNC. She presented Julia's case and got some interesting information and suggestions. She is going to start by making a change in a medication that may be aggravating the situation. If that doesn't work, she has some other ideas up her sleeve. She was very pleased with the way Julia's lungs sounded. They appear to be working quite fine now. Good thing the windows are not open or the neighbors might start complaining.

Mommy and Daddy gave Julia a bath this evening. Mommy showed Julia her reflection in the mirror, but she wasn't too interested yet. Even though she weighed in at 7 lbs 7 oz, there isn't much to her once we get her clothes off. She can be quite slippery too when she gets wet.

Ronan had a good day with Nurse Dawn. He gained some weight last night and is close to six pounds. Last night's gain was probably real weight, but the night before he had a large gain possibly caused by the IV fluids. Nurse Dawn worked with him on his special bottle, and he did very well with it today. They are going to do some tests to find out if there are any enzymes they can give him to help him absorb more fats. Daddy went to visit after work, and he found Ronan wide-awake. He was very interested in looking around the room. He also was interested in looking at Daddy.

135 **November 9, 2006**

We had a busy day today. Julia went in for her eye exam. Although she was unhappy during it, there was good news. Her eyes are more mature now, and she won't have to return for four to six months. Daddy met Mommy at the hospital and sat with Julia in the waiting room while Mom spent some time with Ronan. Julia is pretty popular at the NICU and had lots of visitors. NNPs David and Elizabeth, Nurses Dawn and Lauren, RT Chris and Cristy (Mom of Ronan and Julia's podmates Dylan and Ryan) all came to see her. Everyone was impressed with the amount of weight she's gained since she went home.

Ronan had a surprise today. It was supposed to be Nurse Dawn's day off, but she was called in to work overtime so he got an extra day with her. He behaved very well for her. He was wide-awake as usual at 7:15 a.m. and stayed up for several hours. He also stayed up for a few hours in the afternoon. Mommy and Daddy actually got to see him with his eyes open. That doesn't happen too often. He gained forty grams last night and they increased his feedings by 1 ml an hour. He now weighs 6 lbs 1 oz.

He was a little uncooperative about giving blood, so they were not able to send in all of his tests. The official ultrasound results came back; and his liver, pancreas, and kidneys all look normal. He also had an eye exam this morning, and although his progress is slow, he is making a little. Instead of one week, they scheduled a two-week follow up. He also had a cuddler spend some time with him. He likes the attention from the ladies.

Just remember that good days happen too!

November 10, 2006, at 10:49 AM EST

I'm so happy to hear that yesterday was such a good day for both kids. It was wonderful to finally get to visit with Julia at home and see her so nice and content to be with you two and her bird pals. She's got such gorgeous eye color now, so I'm thrilled that her exam went well and she gets to just grow and grow. She's doing so great, and Ronan is coming along—the big boy now up over 6 lbs! I know that bad days happen and sometimes they seem to pile up, but remember that there are really good days too to even them out. Better yet, the good days will keep getting more and more frequent, and (with some luck) the bad days will get fewer and fewer. Yeah! I'll see you Saturday for a nice walk (if the weather cooperates).

Amber

136 November 11, 2006

Julia had another good day. She took a walk with Mommy and Amber and little Jack. It was a fine day with temps in the seventies, so she spent plenty of time outside, and yes, Mina, we had a hat for her.

Ronan is gaining weight. He gained another seventy grams last night and is starting to fill in quite nicely. We really enjoyed our visit with him this afternoon. He was alert and interested in what was going on around him. It was probably the most alert we've ever seen him. He was looking at everything and even catching our eyes. He was very interested in sucking on his paci and became agitated when it fell out of his mouth. Nurse Tracey said she spent a lot of time this morning standing near the crib holding his paci for him. Mommy practiced with him using his special bottle. Unfortunately, his As and Bs seem to be getting worse, not better. We need to figure that part out before he can come home. We do feel it's getting close to that day though. Even Dr. Wood is impressed with his progress this week, and she demands a lot out of her patients. Thanks again to Nurse Amy who is watching Julia while we visit Ronan. We really do appreciate it a lot.

137 November 12, 2006

Ronan had a minor setback. His As and Bs were getting more severe, and they decided to put him back on the nasal cannula. They started at two liters but have moved it back down to one liter. Nurse Carol is taking care of him today. She has not had him for several months, but she cared for him quite frequently in the beginning. Nurse Dawn is with her trainee today, but she came by to visit a few times. Ronan really perks up when he hears her voice.

Julia is staying with Daddy today while Mommy visits Ronan. Julia continues to be quite the wiggle worm. Last night we swaddled her in a blanket and put her at the top of the crib. We have the mattress raised to help with her reflux. Whenever we got up to feed her, she was at the bottom of the crib with one sock, no blanket, and her gown pushed up to her neck. Of course, her brother is a wiggle worm too. His crib at the hospital is smaller, but he managed to move ninety degrees from where he was placed originally.

138 November 13, 2006

Both kids had good nights. Julia is keeping us on our toes, but she is a good girl with her feedings. Fortunately, we are only up with her twice each night. Unfortunately, she has a nasty habit of spitting up large quantities of milk all over us. Lately, Mommy has gotten the worst of it.

Ronan had a good evening. He has not had any As and Bs since midnight, and he gained five grams last night. Every Monday they check his blood to see if the damage to the liver is being reversed. They can measure this by looking at the level of his bilirubin. Despite the small amount of TPN he received this week, his bilirubin is down by almost half this week. It is still high, but certainly going in the right direction. As his bilirubin levels go down, the yellow color he has been sporting will start to fade.

I was a little concerned about his two nights without weight gain right as they are weaning him off his TPN. Nurse Dawn said they'll definitely keep an eye on his weight. He gained a huge amount the past few days, so she doesn't anticipate he will continue to gain large amounts each night. She does think he would benefit from some enzymes to help him absorb fats, but they are still waiting for his lab results. The plan is to slowly wean him off TPN over the next twenty-four to thirty-six hours.

Ronan is alert, and his best time seems to be early in the mornings. He looks at us and notices other activity in the pod. I guess if anything good is coming out of his extended stay, it's the stimulation he gets during the day. Of course, both kids know how to sleep with noise. We could fire a cannon off next to Julia when she is sleeping, and she would not stir. Mommy and Daddy are learning how to wake up, feed Julia, and then go back to sleep one second after their heads hit the pillow. In fact, some nights Daddy has no idea that he got up, changed, fed, and wrote everything down in detail in her log.

Thanksgiving is coming up, and it will be a pretty quiet day for us. One of us will visit Ronan in the hospital and then we will have some dinner. Luckily Nurse Dawn will spend turkey day with our boy. I promised Ronan that we will celebrate New Year's Eve at home.

139 **November 14, 2006**

Ronan is going downstairs for his swallow study today. They want to make sure everything is going where it should before they are able to start him on regular bottle-feeding. He only had one A and B today and gained twenty grams overnight.

Julia, Mommy, and Daddy are getting used to their routine and would love to have the little brother come home and join them soon.

I'll cross my fingers

November 14, 2006, at 05:02 PM EST

With luck, by the time you read this post, Ronan will have been cleared, and all his innards will be moving everything in the proper direction. He still has much growing to do, so if things are a bit off, that would be expected, but he's come so far . . . so good job, Ronan! Tell him to hurry it up so that he can come home and Julia can tell him about all her lovely walks with Mommy (not that she opens her eyes to look around . . . little sleepyhead loves her walks, huh?) You two parents are doing great, and look how well both kids are doing because of your love and attention and worry!

Amber

140 November 15, 2006

How many adults does it take to give a 7.5 pound baby a bath? Mom and Dad bathed Julia last night. She enjoyed it at first but tired of it before we were finished. She desperately wanted to put her head under the water, but we thought that was a bad idea. Boy, wet babies are slippery.

Ronan had a good night. He was very alert and awake this morning as is his custom. He has not had any As and Bs since midnight and gained fifteen grams last night. He now weighs 2,930 grams which is 6 lbs 8 oz. It is amazing how much we look forward to the daily weight reports. It's our favorite part of the day, second, of course to our daily visits. The nurse took a picture last night of Ronan without his cannula. We hope he'll stay off it for good now.

I talked to the OT about his swallow study. She thought he did very well with it. He has a little bit of reflux to his nose but did not aspirate any milk to his lungs. They tested him in both semiupright and sideline positions. The "old" way of feeding babies is semiupright. Now they feed babies (at least preemies) in a sideline position. The nurse (or parent) crosses his/her legs and places the baby on his side parallel to the raised thigh. The head is raised slightly since it is supported by the leg. It seems that Ronan was not very happy when they tried to test him in a semiupright position. He has never fed this way, and he wasn't about to start. He was flinging his head around and actually spit back out some milk. The OT said she is comfortable trying the slow-flow nipple with Ronan now. This is one step better than his "special" bottle. She'll try to feed him with the slow flow at least once a day during the week.

We've been keeping the CarePages kind of sterile and factual, but I feel the need to talk a little bit about my thoughts and feelings. I've got the normal new-Mom fears that my kids will stop breathing, get sick, get injured; but I won't go on for pages with the rest of my fears. On top of that, I don't know the full effects that coming into this world fifteen weeks early will have on them. It is not likely I'll know anytime soon either. It could be as minor as some developmental delays to which they will catch up as they get older, or it could be much worse than that. At this point, Julia's worst problem seems to be her lungs. I know that they will get better as time passes. She may have asthma or allergies. She may have eye problems or not grow as much as the average kid. My guess is that Julia will not have serious long-term problems.

On the other hand, Ronan is a question mark. There is still a chance he could pull through without any major long-term effects. However, I worry about how the things they did to keep him alive will affect him down the road. He received TPN nutrition long-term, ventilator support long-term and high doses of blood pressure medication. He's had multiple invasive surgeries, and he doesn't always remember or isn't always able to keep breathing and/or keep his heart beating fast enough.

In addition, there seems to be some question as to why he is not absorbing all the nutrients he needs from his intestines although they are doing some tests to pinpoint how they can best help him absorb more nutrients until his intestine has grown enough to overcome the trauma it has faced. The doctors do tell us that if a baby has to have Necrotizing enterocolitis, it is better to have it as a twenty-five weeker than as a full-term baby. Ronan has a lot more time to catch up and grow the kind of intestine he needs to sustain him than a full-term baby would have.

I worry that he, unlike Julia, may have something more severe than "developmental delays." The truth is that there is not much I can do about it right now. When he gets home, I can help by making sure he is stimulated and give him lots of attention. Studies have been done showing that if parents work with these children enough early on, it can help preemies overcome some of their obstacles. I need to make the commitment to do everything I can for him and be understanding and patient with any long-term problems he might have. If I am good to and patient with him, he will learn to be the same to me.

I've been lucky with the weather since Julia got home. We've had a lot of sixty and seventy degree days. When I am working and there is a sixty or seventy degree day in the fall, I often miss the whole thing. When I am at home with the baby, I can go for a walk whenever I want as long as I work it around the feeding and doctor schedule. I take her out for a few hours every day that it is nice. Most days I walk down to the park with her or walk along the trails. When I go to the park, I turn into a nervous teenager/social moron with the other parents I meet. It gets kind of lonely at home with an infant and I don't have much social interaction. I can't go to the store or the mall or any public place for fear of exposing her to germs and all of my friends work full time.

At first I didn't really want to talk to the other parents at the park. I've heard a lot of people at work complain that stay-at-home moms aren't very friendly to working moms, so I've been a little hesitant. In addition, I get butterflies in my stomach as I approach the park. I am really afraid to go up and start a conversation with someone. It is worse when they are standing around in groups and all seem to know each other. I had the same problem in graduate school. I used to get very nervous during class breaks. I really wanted to join the conversation, but I couldn't bring myself to make the move. It is so ironic that my brother's main joy in life is going up to strangers and talking to them. I wonder why I'm not like him.

We think Julia may have colic. She cries all the time when she is not sleeping or eating. The articles we have read say that the cause is unknown; and there is not much that can be done for colic other than holding, rubbing, and burping the baby, putting her in her swing, or giving her a pacifier. Basically, that's everything we already do. The fun part is that most babies outgrow it by eight or nine months. Joy.

Dad wasn't feeling well today and didn't want to expose Ronan to anything, so I went to see him again today. We had a very nice visit. The OT supervised while I gave Ronan 20 ml of milk with a normal bottle and a slow flow nipple. He took 15 ml for her at 2:00 p.m. He has some work to do before he becomes an expert bottle-feeder. He has a habit of leaving his mouth open and sticking his tongue out. They think that he started doing it to counter his floppy airway, and it became a habit. It is kind of sad when we touch the tip of his tongue. It feels like sandpaper. Anyway, his tongue gets in the way when he sucks the bottle. The OT says that as a result of the tongue, he doesn't get a strong suck, and he is doing a lot of work, but not getting a lot of result. However, he does make up for it in enthusiasm. This baby wants to suck all the time. He is dying to be bottle-fed. When he is not sucking the pacifier, he sucks anything that gets near him—washcloths, the fabric on his swing, the Neopuff, and when there is nothing nearby, he just sucks at the air.

I was really excited about getting a picture of Ronan without his cannula. His face looks so different without it. The nurse took a few pictures of me holding him, but he looks very yellow from the elevated bilirubin when he is next to me. I then tried to take some pictures of him held at arm's length. That wasn't working out, either. My next try was to prop him up in the crib against a blanket and take pictures of him that way. He kept falling over to the side. I finally got him propped up with blankets and started snapping. As soon as I clicked the camera, he blinked. The next time, I would poke his tongue back in his mouth, but he'd open his mouth and stick his tongue out again as soon as I clicked the camera. I took about twenty pictures and was able to find a handful that was pretty good. Ed really likes the one picture he calls "Silly Ronan." He has a silly grin on his face and his tongue is sticking out at the camera. This was a popular picture on the grandparent front too. Mina printed it out for her fridge and says hello to Silly Ronan every day.

141 November 16, 2006

Julia had an appointment today with the pulmonologist at UNC. It was a little crazy today because they are having an auction, and the lobby is a madhouse. It makes me really uncomfortable to have my ex-twenty-five weeker with chronic lung disease (who is still on oxygen) out in that kind of atmosphere during flu season.

The pulmonologist was impressed with Julia's growth. She weighs 7 lbs 13 oz and is 21.5 inches long. However, she is still a little concerned about her breathing. Her lungs sound good, but the doctor can tell that she is still laboring at her breathing from watching her belly and her slight head bob. She may be on oxygen a little longer than we originally thought. The pulmonologist says we need to be really careful during the winter and flu season. We don't want her to have to work too hard to breathe. We will leave her on the .2 liters, and when the time comes, we will wean her very slowly. I guess she can't get away with that little trick Ronan pulled. The pulmonologist put my mind at ease about the spit-ups and coughing. She said that reflux is very common, and she is not concerned because Julia is still growing. That is pretty much what everyone else has told us too, but it is good to hear it again. She is going to try her on a new reflux medication. It'll be fun cutting the tablet in half, crushing it, and mixing it with water. I saw the nurse do that with Ronan's medication last night. On the other hand, it'd be great if it made her feel better. She often seems very uncomfortable after a meal.

There was no way I was leaving the hospital without stopping by to see Ronan. I can't imagine the NICU is any less healthy than the lobby and the clinic waiting area. I brought Julia into the front hall of the NICU. NNP Elizabeth, Dr. Wood, and RT Chris came by to say hello. They were very impressed with how big she has gotten. Dr. Wood came over to see Julia and see how big Ronan should be. Elizabeth was kind enough to watch Julia while I went in quickly to say hello to Ronan. Ronan has an unfortunate choice of bedding and outfits today. He has a yellow quilt under him, a yellow blanket over him and a yellow outfit on him, so he looks very jaundiced today. Good thing Nurse Dawn is not here to see it! My fault, I have been meaning to take that yellow outfit home.

He is exactly the same weight as yesterday which means he is almost a pound and a half less than Julia. He has only had one minor spell since midnight. The OT worked with him on his bottle-feedings again today. He took 14 ml but spit up half of it. Speaking of spit-ups, Julia and Elizabeth were covered in formula when I returned. I'm so sorry, Elizabeth!

142 November 17, 2006

Ronan had a good night and is very happy to have Nurse Amy caring for him today. However, he lost twenty grams last night, and his weight is basically flat for the week. We are worried that he will need to go back on TPN. Apparently his intestine just cannot absorb the fats he needs now. Hopefully this will resolve itself as he gets bigger. The tests that were sent to the Mayo clinic indicated his vitamin levels are within range so enzymes probably won't help him. Once again we are very worried about him. He needs to grow so TPN is the only choice, but the risk to his liver makes it a difficult one.

Julia had another restless night. We think her fortified formula and heavy vitamin regimen are contributing to her discomfort. No matter how much sleep we are missing, we are thrilled to have her home with us and cannot wait until her brother joins us.

143 November 18, 2006

Ronan lost another ten grams last night. We are still very concerned that his body just cannot absorb the nutrients he needs to grow. We think he will need to go back on TPN on a more permanent basis until his system can process the fats he needs. Otherwise he seems to be doing well. He is working very hard at his bottle-feedings and really has the swing of it now. He is also very alert and interested in what is going on around him. Mommy visited him last night and said he was a sleepyhead for the most part, but he did wake up a few times to say hello.

Julia had a great night. Though she still grunts and groans a lot during the night, her spit-ups seem to be fewer and less extreme. However, she just nailed Mommy and her stuffed elephant a little while ago.

144 November 19, 2006

Ronan gained ten grams last night. We're going to have to have a long talk with the attending physician tomorrow. The current plan is obviously not working, and we need to develop a new plan. Otherwise, he is doing fine. Mommy visited him today, and he took 20 ml of milk from the bottle. Then he and Mommy enjoyed a long snuggle.

Daddy stayed home with Julia. He was out raking leaves while Julia was on her new baby monitor. The birds made more noise on the monitor than she did. We've been trying to give Julia tummy time like all the reading material suggests, but she doesn't seem to like it very much. She always gets fussy and cries when we put her on her tummy. In fact, she appeared to roll over last night when placed on her tummy. We're not sure if it was an accident because it seems a little too early for rolling over. I guess we'll have to see if she does it again.

145 November 20, 2006

We are very happy to report that Ronan gained fifty grams last night. Monday is bilirubin day, and his bilirubin is exactly the same as last week. We'd really prefer to see it go down, but at least it didn't go up. Right now he is taking a snooze in his swing while the NICU nurses attend to recently born triplets.

Julia is going to see the pediatrician today at 2:00 p.m. Right now she is snoozing in her bouncy chair.

146 November 20, 2006

Daddy visited with Ronan tonight. He had a great day. He was held by three different nurses, two cuddlers, and Daddy. He was alert and interested in what the new triplets were up to in his pod. He also took a bottle for Daddy and is really getting the hang of it. Good boy, Ronan. Daddy also had a long talk with Dr. Wood. Ronan is still struggling with his weight, and she'd recommend putting him on long-term TPN to supplement his regular feedings. They will insert a central arterial line (called a Broviac) into him so Mommy and Daddy can give him the TPN at home. Though it sounds daunting and scary, if this is what it takes to get our boy home, then we will do it. We know he will thrive at home with his family, and all the positive stimulation and attention.

Julia went to the pediatrician. The pediatrician is very pleased with her progress, especially in the weight department. Her weight is 8 lbs 4 oz. Nurse Amy came over for a visit and joined Mommy and Daddy for dinner while enjoying a visit with her little "bubby." Julia really seems to perk up when Amy is around. Thanks, Amy, for taking the time to visit. Overall, things seem to be settling in here though we know that it will all get tossed upside-down when the boy comes home. Then again, our lives have been upside-down since Friday, July 7, at 8:30 a.m. We also will do anything to have Ronan home. We are willing to stay up all night taking care of both of them if we can finally all be together.

147 November 21, 2006

We just gave Julia a bath. She seemed to take it better than usual. Nurse Kerry suggested we put a cloth diaper over the parts that weren't being washed to keep the heat in, and that seemed to do the trick. We gave her a fresh nasal cannula and a fresh pulsox. While we were switching out the nasal cannula, we snapped a few pictures since we never get to see her face. Although compared to how much the CPAP and ventilators covered, we do get to see most of her face with the cannula. As we were taping the cannula, she grabbed my finger and started using it as a paci. She has an impressive amount of suction for a small baby.

Dad went and got the real paci to try to avoid baby meltdown. Amber and Gene coined that phrase, but we like it a lot. Baby meltdown is what happens when we feed the baby on demand. Rather than feeding her exactly every three or four hours, we wait until she is ready. Unfortunately, by the time she tells us she is ready, it is already too late. She has already progressed to baby meltdown stage.

It is difficult to change her, put on her bib, give her medications, and start feeding during baby meltdown. As soon as we get the bottle in, baby meltdown ends and baby feeding begins. It'll be daunting when we experience double baby meltdown.

Today was the end of Ronan's seven-day test period. He received seven days of 25 percent TPN and gained 345 grams and seven days of 100 percent formula and gained sixty grams. At this point, we are comfortable with Dr. Wood's recommendation to start partial TPN again. They have tried everything else and nothing has worked. Ronan will not thrive if he can't grow. If giving him TPN is the only way to make him grow, we have to go down that path.

The surgeons called to get consent to insert the central cardiac line or Broviac for Ronan's TPN. It is much safer to use this longer term because an IV line can be too easily pulled out. Ronan is on the surgery schedule tomorrow as an add-on case. It could be done at bedside, but the surgeons feel more comfortable doing it in the OR. We hope they are able to fit him in tomorrow before the holiday. Otherwise, we are facing another delay of at least five days, and we hate to see any more delays. Please wish him good luck.

You guys are the masters of daunting and scary!

November 21, 2006, at 10:36 AM EST

With all you've been through, doing that TPN at home is going to be easy. You have had amazing strength and courage throughout this ordeal, and once home, these guys are going to thrive—as is obvious by Julia's plumping up!

Keep up the good work, guys! Way to grow, Julia! Keep at it, Ronan!
Aimee

November 22, 2006

Ronan lost five grams last night but did not have any As and Bs. They stopped his feeds in anticipation of his surgery. The nurses report he is not happy about that. We hope they can fit him on the surgery schedule today. Otherwise he will have to wait until after the holiday.

Tomorrow we will bring Julia with us to the NICU for a little family reunion. We have a sleep room reserved so all four of us can spend a few hours together. The kids have not seen each other for almost a month. We know it is too early for them to pay too much attention to each other, but we're looking forward to it anyway.

Giving thanks. This Thanksgiving means a lot to us. For the last four months we have had many ups and many downs, but we always held out hope even when the future looked bleak. At this time of the year, we give thanks for each day we have with Ronan and Julia. Each night when we give Julia her feedings at 2:00 a.m., we acknowledge there is nothing else we would rather do (other than feeding both kids). Each visit to Ronan is special to us as we watch him get bigger, knowing he is coming home soon. We have had many reasons in the past to give thanks, but it all pales in comparison to this year. This really puts what is important and what matters most into perspective.

Happy Thanksgiving... Ed, Nicole, Ronan, Julia, Alexander, and Zebulon

149 November 22, 2006

Update from Ed: Ronan was just getting back from surgery when Daddy arrived for a visit. Even though he was coming off general anesthesia, he was alert and interested in what was going on in the pod. I guess the triplets are fascinating to watch. The Broviac line was inserted successfully with no complications. In fact, the dressing on his incision is in the shape of a turkey. Get it—the dressing is a turkey. Ha-ha.

Prayers for Ronan for surgery

November 22, 2006, at 08:18 AM EST

It sounds good to have a real concrete comparison of with and without TPN weight gain to see what works better. Praying that the TPN doesn't hurt little Ronan in the future, the surgery goes well, and he can say good-bye to TPN sooner this way all around. It is a tough decision, but you have all the nurses' and doctors' support and advice and the home team pulling for you. Hope you are feeling our support!

Have a great Thanksgiving! I'll be missing the tofu turkey this year!

Love, Sue

150 November 23, 2006

Happy Thanksgiving, everyone! Today is our big family day. We arrived at the hospital around 11:00 a.m. It was unnaturally quiet and peaceful in the lobby. Nurse Dawn is back from her time with her family, and she bought Ronan a new outfit. It has chocolate brown stripes and looks very good with his complexion. This morning, the babies all made turkey handprints to celebrate Thanksgiving. Ronan's turkey handprint was accompanied by a fabulous photo of him looking awake and alert. The surgery didn't slow him down at all.

Thanks to all the staff who is working on the Thanksgiving holiday. They don't get to sneak out early like some employees do on Thanksgiving. They are in it for twelve and a half hours just like they are every day they work. The mood was festive, and there was a potluck for the staff. There was also a Thanksgiving meal for patients and parents of pediatric patients.

Shortly after we arrived, we rolled Ronan into the sleep room for his visit. This is actually the first time he has ever been in the sleep room. He appeared to enjoy the ride over, once he realized he wasn't going down to surgery. At first, both kids were absolutely zonked out. We held them up to each other and tried to get them to wake up. That didn't work so we deposited both of them in Ronan's crib and tried to get them to hold hands. Ronan eventually woke up, but he was more interested in finding his paci; observing his new surroundings; and looking at Mom, Dad, and Dawn than he was in hanging out with his sister. We got them snuggled up next to each other and snapped a bunch of pictures. I made a poor choice of color for Julia, and she looked a little washed out in a pale pink sleeper next to bronze Ronan. Last week, one of the cuddlers kept talking about Ronan's tan. I'm not sure she understands the concept of jaundice. Even if she doesn't understand that, how does she think he got a tan if he's never been outside? She was an older lady, and her enthusiasm made up for her strange comments.

Julia did wake up for a few minutes when she was ready to eat. I had left the sleep room for a few minutes, and I could hear her baby meltdown through two doors on my way back. During her meltdown, Julia managed to whack Ronan a few times in the face. I fear this won't be the last time. At the same time, Ronan was trying to suck milk out of Julia's outfit in his never-ending quest to feed from a bottle. Finally it was feeding time, and Mommy fed Ronan his bottle while Julia took hers from Dad. Ronan took 16 ml.

The plan for Ronan is to give him continuous feedings at night through his g-tube and bolis feedings throughout the day. Bolis feeds are the opposite of continuous feedings. That way we can prepare him for the fact that he won't be getting continuous feedings forever. GI will come early next week to look things over and make sure it is OK to start this new plan. He also needs to work on his As and Bs before he can come home. That's all the news from Pod C, sleep room 1, and Weston Pointe.

151 **November 24, 2006**

It's almost 10:00 p.m., and Julia is finally quiet. I left poor Dad at home with Julia when I went to the hospital to see Ronan, and he was a little frazzled when I got back. It is sometimes tough to be home with the birds and Julia when they are all screaming. I know this because I feel that way most days when they all have meltdown at the same time. Julia is having some quality awake time right now. She loves the poster of the Sebastiani Vineyards that hangs over the couch. She'll gaze at it adoringly for several minutes at a time. Dad even held her up so she could touch it. Whatever works!

Ronan had a good day today. He has not had any As and Bs in two days. His weight did go down today about two ounces, but that was to be expected as he lost the extra fluid he accumulated during his surgery. He is doing well with his bottle-feedings. Mom gave him 20 ml at 5:00 p.m., and he sucked it down in no time. He spent the next two hours asking for more. If he'll be patient, he'll get to drink more from the bottle in a few days. He was a little fussy today whenever Nurse Dawn had to pay attention to her other baby. I have news for him—when he gets home there will be two babies here too. He will need to learn the lesson of sharing at an early age.

152 **November 26, 2006**

Julia had a tough night. She was cranky and awake off and on all night long. She is having some issues with her plumbing, so she is not happy. A daily dose of prune juice doesn't seem to be helping much. She slept a lot of the day, but was up to visit with Lori, Sue, and Terry this evening.

She reminds me of that cartoon of the screaming baby with the huge open mouth, a curled tongue, and tonsils. It makes so much more sense to me now.

Daddy went to visit Ronan today at the hospital. Apparently he was cranky for Nurse Amy in the afternoon but settled down when Daddy arrived. Daddy fed him 12 ml, but he spit most of it back up. He has a tough time with his bottle-feedings since he is already receiving feeds through his g-tube. The plan is to feed him with bottles during the day starting Monday and then give him continuous feedings at night through the g-tube and TPN at night. There is even talk that with the progress he is making, he could come home the week of December 4. Of course, this is all speculation at this point. He needs to behave and show us that he is strong enough not to have any As and Bs. It has been three days since his last one which was caused by a formula spit-up. Could it be that we may be near the end of this saga? Special thanks today to Nurses Amy and Amie for making it a nice day for Ronan.

153 November 26, 2006

Ronan gained weight for the second night in a row. He weighs seven pounds. He is still A and B free. He's been cranky again today and is trying everyone's patience. Hopefully when he starts on his bolis feeds, he'll feel fuller and not be so fussy. Let's hope for a good bilirubin read tomorrow. By the way, it turns out his bilirubin actually went up slightly last week. It didn't stay the same as we reported earlier.

Julia is having a good day, but we haven't hit fussy time yet. The tag on her bib kept her busy for several hours this afternoon. She kept trying to lick it. Julia and Mommy went for a walk with Amber, Jack, and Claire. Surprisingly enough, Julia actually stayed awake for a little while during the walk.

154 November 27, 2006

Ronan had another good night of weight gain. He is now an established member of the three-kilogram club, weighing in at 3,250 grams or approximately 7 lbs 2 oz. His direct bilirubin level is slightly down from last week and comes in at 6.7. The level should really be closer to 1, but it will be a very long time before it gets there. His other labs all came back at an acceptable level including the sweat test for cystic fibrosis. Unfortunately, they did not start the bolis feeds today. The new plan is to stop his continuous feedings at 6:00 a.m. tomorrow and start him on his bolis feeds at 8:00 a.m.

Julia attracted a lot of attention out on her walk today. Everyone kept stopping to tell me she was cute and tiny. Somehow she looks like a giant to me. Nurse Amy came over and initiated some playtime on Julia's activity mat. Julia actually spent about twenty minutes of fairly happy play interacting with a menagerie of stuffed animals and baby development toys and kicking up a storm with her legs.

155 November 28, 2006

Everybody had a good night. Ronan continues to gain weight with the help of the evil TPN. He weighs 3,300 grams or 7 lbs 4 oz. He began bottle-feeding during the day this morning. Apparently he was not too pleased about the doctors' stopping his g-tube feedings at 6:00 a.m. He let Nurse Donna know he was displeased. Our boy is getting a bit of an independent streak. He knows what he wants and will settle for nothing less. There is still talk that he will be coming home next week if he behaves himself. He has not had an A and B spell in six days. The plan is still for the GI team to take over his long-term care. We never thought we would get to the day when "coming home" was mentioned in the same breath as "Ronan."

Julia also had a good night. It's amazing how a little dark Karo syrup can get things back on track. Sweetie pie really enjoyed her visit with Nurse Amy last night. She was like a different kid. We are glad she had fun with her friend.

I have a new outlook on the park. Walking in the park is not about me. It is about me and Julia. I need to enjoy my time with my daughter, so whatever else happens is irrelevant. I took this new attitude with me to the park today. We are having another streak of good weather, and I headed down to the park in a very good mood.

I think I have a touch of seasonal affective disorder, and I'm normally kind of bummed after daylight savings time ends each fall. When I am working, it sometimes is dark when I get there and dark when I leave.

Julia seemed to be in a good mood too. I cranked up the iPod and enjoyed our walk. I got to the park and sat in the sunshine and read my book and chatted with Julia. A couple of people actually came up to me. My neighbor came to say hello, and we chatted for a few minutes. Then another mother and her friend came by and introduced themselves. It turns out that the mother had a former twenty-seven weeker who is now around five. We chatted for a while, and she had some comforting things to say.

157 November 29, 2006

There is no new news about Ronan's GI stay today. The NNP has been paging the GI doctor all day, and her calls have not been returned. We'd really like to get some information on the plan for Ronan so we can make our own plans.

158 November 30, 2006

Ronan has had a very busy morning. He has not had any more As and Bs. His A and B test period is over at midnight tonight. If a baby does not have an As and Bs within eight days, they are very unlikely to have another.

All babies that go home from the NICU have to pass the car seat test. They have to be able to sit in the car seat for the amount of time it will take the parents to get home without having any problems. Ronan passed with flying colors.

Ronan also had another eye exam this morning. His right eye is almost matured, but his left eye is slightly worse. The good news is that the doctor doesn't seem too concerned about it since she doesn't want to see him for three weeks. Ronan took 45 ml from his bottle this morning and did not spit up. He is being very good for Nurse Dawn. Dawn will show Dad how to take care of the g-tube tonight, and she'll show Mom tomorrow. We'll have to learn to keep it clean, watch for problems around the site, and feed him through it. They still have not heard back from GI.

Julia is awake and alert this morning. After her morning bottle, she has been looking around at everything. Sometimes it is hard to tell what has caught her eye.

Wow What a Great Day

November 30, 2006, at 11:22 AM EST

Here's what I think—when Julia got together with Ronan on Thanksgiving she told him what a great time she was having at home, and he decided he better shape up and get there himself! Big smiles.

Mary Ellen

Thanks for the update

November 30, 2006, at 09:21 AM EST

Thank you so much for the constant updates. I know this is so you will remember this very special time, but it's great for us who like to keep tabs on Julia and Ronan's well-being. The new pictures are great, and it is so nice to "see" Amy. We have heard so much about this very special person . . . Take care and get prepared, sounds like there will be two little ones at home soon.

Ellen

159 December 1, 2006

Ronan has a tentative discharge date of Friday, Dec 8. Daddy met with the GI doctor. They will monitor his calories and adjust everything as he grows. A home healthcare aide will come to the house to help out from time to time. Mommy and Daddy will be taught to feed him through the g-tube/Mic-Key button, hang his TPN, and manage his Broviac. Daddy learned how to use Ronan's g-tube last night. It is not exactly rocket science. They are working on weaning him to where he will receive TPN and continuous feedings at night. He will bottle-feed during the day. He did very well on his bottles for Dawn and Daddy. He also slept for almost the entire night. He is such a good boy, and we think he is ready to come home and join us.

Julia had a good night. She only woke up once for a feeding and was in good spirits today. However she has her RSV shot this morning, so she may not be happy for long. Ronan has his too, but a little shot is nothing to our brave man. He laughs at needles at this point.

I stopped at work on the way to the hospital to get the latest updates and virus protection for my laptop. My remote access does not work unless this is done periodically, and for some reason it won't let me do this at home. Ed had a meeting and was going to be a few minutes late, so one of my coworkers volunteered to sit with Julia while I did this. I sneaked in the back door and tried to take care of business quietly, so I didn't have to say hello to all my coworkers. I know my dad would call that antisocial behavior, but the alternative was having my time with Ronan cut short. We are only allowed to stay until 7:00 p.m., and I hate giving up part of that time. While my laptop was updating, I peeked out the window a few times, and it seemed like there was a steady line of people who stopped by to see what was going on. Everyone loves babies, and the CarePages are very popular at my office.

When I got to the hospital, I had to run into the parents' room for a minute, and I saw someone talking on a cell phone. This has been a bone of contention for us since day one. The patients and visitors at the hospitals go to great lengths to flout the rules. There are always patients (sometimes very sick ones) and visitors smoking in front of the hospital right next to the No Smoking, No Se Fuma signs, and there are always people in the parents' room talking on cell phones despite the No Cell Phones Allowed signs. There were only a few of these signs when we started using the room, but Ed has tacked up plenty of extra ones.

I politely suggested that the cell phone user go downstairs to make her call. In a snotty tone of voice, she said, "There is someone here who has an attitude, so I guess I need to get off the phone." We were told that cell phones interfere with the monitoring equipment that they use for the babies. I was shocked that someone who obviously had a baby in the NICU would be that callous about her baby or the babies of others. She really pushed my buttons, and we had some words. The man with her interrupted and told me that they've had a baby in the NICU for a long time. I told him that I have too and they ought to know better. It was very unpleasant. I can't wait until we don't have to go to that place with all the inconsiderate, ignorant people anymore.

160 December 1, 2006

Julia the Giant weighed 8 lbs 13 oz at today's doctor appointment. We can't believe how big she is getting. The doctor is very happy with the way she is growing. She also is very pleased with the way Julia's lungs sound. Julia got her Synagis shot and one other shot today. As soon as the needles went in her skin, her face turned red, the tongue curled slightly, and she started crying. Her boo-boos were quickly covered with bright blue, bright orange, and Elmo characters. Fortunately, the crying didn't last long, and after the mandatory twenty-minute waiting period we were allowed to leave.

Midnight came and went and Ronan did not have any As and Bs. He gained twenty-five grams and weighs 7 lbs 5 1/2 oz. The doctors haven't been happy with his weight gain the last few days so they switched him from twenty-four-calorie formula back to twenty-six-calorie formula. As a result, he had a few spit-ups during his bottle-feeding today. Poor Dawn had several stains on her scrubs by the time I got there. Ronan took 40 ml for Mom but did not spit up for that feeding.

After the feeding, Mom learned all about the care of the g-tube. After the oxygen and monitor that Julia brought home, this seems like a breeze. I'm much less nervous this time. We'll see if I still feel that way after the TPN training. Before I left for the evening, we gave Ronan a quick bath. He seemed to enjoy it. If he keeps behaving himself, he might give Mom the best birthday present ever.

161 December 3, 2006

Ronan has gained weight the last two nights and now weighs 7 lbs 9 oz. He is still learning how to feed by bottle and had two minor feeding-related episodes last night. One was an apnea where his oxygen saturation went down to 60 percent after his feedings—it should be in the nineties, but he brought himself out of it quickly. He also had a bradycardia last night after a feeding where his heart rate dipped, but he came out of that one fairly easily too. During rounds, the doctors will discuss whether this will affect his plan. We're hoping it won't since they were both minor and both feeding related. An episode in the middle of the night while he was sleeping, with no apparent cause, would be more serious.

Julia is Julia. She eats, sleeps, cries, looks at walls and ceilings, and occasionally looks alert. Sometimes she'll have an involuntary twitch of her muscles, and it looks like she is trying to put out a small smile.

162 December 4, 2006

Ronan had a bad spell last night while he was asleep. That is the worst kind. The nurse had to do vigorous stimulation to get him to breathe again. He also had some spit-up issues this morning. Unfortunately, this means they will need to start the eight-day A and B countdown again. We are very worried about his development. He is already a micropreemie with the likelihood of developmental delays. Leaving him in a hospital bed for hours at a stretch with minimal stimulation or interaction is not going to help him catch up. It is really time for him to come home with his family where kids typically grow and thrive. Once again, he has a nurse today who has never had him before. This means he will spend a lot of time in bed with no interaction.

Julia had a rather large spit-up last night. She coated Daddy around 2:30 a.m. and did the same to Mommy later in the morning. On the lighter side, the staff in the NICU has come up with lots of names for our boy. There is Ronan the Barbarian, Late Night with Ronan, and the Ronan Catholic Church. The pope name was rather clever. He has a strange-looking hat that looks sort of like the pope's hat.

Since today's nurse didn't know Ronan and I forgot to ask, she didn't mention his bilirubin results. Nurse Dawn was kind enough to look up his bilirubin test on her day off and e-mail us the results. His direct bilirubin went down this week to 5.6. That is a small piece of good news. Once again we are aiming for something in the neighborhood of 1. Since he is on TPN, we don't expect to have it happen quickly. However, small, incremental improvements are always appreciated.

163 December 5, 2006

Both kids had a good night. Ronan had no episodes last night. He gained forty grams and now weighs 3,470 grams or 7 lbs 10.5 oz. Nurse Amy is taking care of him today. She fed him a bottle this morning, and he took about 45 ml with a small spit-up. We talked to NNP Elizabeth last night about his discharge date. He needs to stay until next Tuesday because of the A and B from Sunday night. He also still needs to be examined by the GI doctors.

On a happier note, Ronan has permission to wander the hospital when he is not on his continuous feeds and TPN. Last night, Mommy took him for a walk around the NICU. They looked at all the pictures painted on the wall and said hello to a few of his friends. By the time they completed the first lap, he was off to dreamland. The nap didn't last too long though. He woke up during their visit to his old stomping grounds in Pod B. He visited with Nurse Amie. We think he has his eye on one of the triplets in there. When Mommy visits tomorrow she will bring the stroller and take him downstairs for a walk in the atrium. If it is warm enough, they will visit the butterfly gardens. He will not be visiting Wendy's.

Julia had fun last night with Nurse Amy. She came to watch her while Mommy and Daddy visited Ronan. As usual, Julia was very happy to have her best friend around for a few hours. Thanks, Amy!

164 December 6, 2006

Ronan had another severe A and B last night while sleeping. His new goal for coming home is next Thursday. NNP Elizabeth and I had a long talk with him and told him that breathing is not optional. He needs to breathe all the time, twenty-four hours a day, and seven days a week.

Mommy and Daddy are meeting with the GI doctor on Friday. We will also be attending classes to learn to care for Ronan's g-tube and Broviac. We are so ready to be done with this.

The big boy gained another eighty grams and is up to 7 lbs 13 oz. That is awfully big for a guy who started at 2 lbs 2 oz.

Julia is Julia. Keep her fed and hold her, and she is a happy girl.

166 December 7, 2006

The twins were born five months ago today. We always think about it at 5:13 p.m. Usually one of us is at the hospital at that time, so it's easy to remember. Also some of the nurses remember that day very well. As we have learned, twins really throw a wrench in the system. Twenty-five week twins cause an explosion, especially with only a few hours notice.

Ronan had a good night. He did a little coughing with a small spit-up, but he didn't have any As and Bs. He gained thirty grams and weighs 3,580 or 7 lbs 14 oz. Nurse Amy is taking care of him today, so we know he is in great hands. Nurse Dawn will also be back tomorrow so Ronan is having a great week. All of his friends are taking good care of him. Daddy will visit his boy this afternoon.

Julia spent a typical night being a little fussy. Daddy is working at home today, and he spent some time with his girl this morning. She saw what Daddy actually does for a living. It is not too interesting, but it keeps Daddy occupied. Daddy also took the opportunity to snap a picture of his cutie during tummy time.

167 December 8, 2006

Mom and Dad met with the GI doctor today to discuss Ronan's plan. She emphasized that we are going to be acting as skilled nurses in caring for Ronan and that it will be a lot of work. We always have to keep in mind during these conversations that doctors have to make sure they explain all scenarios, even the unlikely ones. Ronan is not a typical TPN patient. He is on a very low level of TPN and is not expected to stay on it forever. We got the feeling during the conversation that the doctor was not necessarily taking this into consideration as she was speaking with us. The doctor said that it normally takes about two weeks for parents to get comfortable with how to do everything. That was a little upsetting because Ronan was supposed to come home next Thursday if he doesn't have any As and Bs. We hope two weeks is for the typical TPN parent because our goal is to beat that by a week. We're going to try to make the most of each day that we visit this coming week to learn as much as we can as fast as we can.

168 December 9, 2006

Mom went to the hospital today to see Ronan. We took a walk around the NICU and looked at all the nursery rhymes on the wall. Then we went downstairs and walked through the Children's Hospital and Neurosciences building. Ronan was fussing before we left, then he looked fascinated, and then he fell asleep. When we returned to Pod C, he opened his eyes and looked a little confused as to where he was. Then he resumed his fussing. Nurse Dawn trained Mom on how to program the feeding pump that will deliver Ronan's continuous feedings for twelve hours each evening after he comes home.

Julia had a quiet day at home with Daddy. She is frustrated because no one will disclose the identity of the baby in the mirror. She sees her every time she goes up the stairs and every time she comes down the stairs.

169 December 10, 2006

Daddy went to visit Ronan today. He was in good spirits for Daddy's visit. He is getting ready to come home. The target date for his discharge is now Thursday. We hope this will be a smooth week for our boy. Daddy learned how to use the feeding pump today that we'll use to give Ronan formula through his g-tube at night. The theory is that he will be able to absorb more nutrients from a continuous/steady feeding at night but still be able to practice the bolis bottle-feeds during the day. He is looking forward to coming home. He has spent more than his fair share of time in the NICU. Mommy and Daddy are also very excited to have him come home.

Julia is having a tough time with her digestion. She is very uncomfortable most of the time and has a lot of reflux. The doctors tell us this is normal even for full-term babies, but it upsets us to watch her in obvious discomfort. Julia helped make Mommy's birthday a very happy day. It was a nice afternoon, and the three of us went for a walk to the park. Next week Ronan will be joining us for our weekend walk.

170 December 11, 2006

Ronan didn't get to take a walk today because he was moved to the isolation room. During a routine swab, he tested positive for Orsa again. Fortunately, this will not affect his scheduled discharge date. If he continues to remain A and B free, he will go home on Thursday.

Ronan's direct bilirubin is down again this week. His reading is 4.9 which is down from 5.6 last week. Once again we have a goal of 1, but don't expect to get there for a long time because the TPN interferes with the liver function.

Ronan gained twenty grams today, but he had a net loss of five grams over the last four nights. I was concerned they might have to increase his TPN to get him to continue to gain weight. However, they are not yet concerned for a couple of reasons. The first is that they have been making a lot of adjustments to his TPN, and it may take awhile for his body to be able to adjust to the new schedule. The second is that they weigh him at night after he has been off the TPN for twelve hours. They recommended that we don't weigh him every day when he gets home. Once or twice a week will give us a more accurate idea of the trend.

Ronan is scheduled for his circumcision tonight. Mom was a little teary eyed when she heard it was going to happen tonight, but the nurse assured her that they put Lidocaine on it to numb it and give him Tylenol afterward in case there is any pain. It is typically not very painful, but he could feel a little sore for a day or two when he urinates.

Julia and Mom went through the pharmacy drive-through today to drop off all of Ronan's prescriptions in preparation for his homecoming. Julia has a pulmonologist appointment tomorrow at UNC. We're going to ask if she still needs the pulsox since she really isn't desatting anymore. However, they will probably suggest we continue to use it until she is off oxygen entirely. Perhaps they will at least let us turn down the oxygen a bit.

Ed is talking to his mom right now, and she asked him who went to the hospital today. He said, "Nicole did, I stayed with Grumpy." She does cry a lot. We hope she'll grow out of that phase soon.

171 December 12, 2006

The Big Guy got clipped last night. Mommy called around 9:30 p.m., and the nurse said he did fine. He was getting ready for bed and did not appear to be uncomfortable at all. Daddy will learn to use the TPN pump this afternoon, and then we should be all set.

Julia is still struggling with her digestion. She spends a good part of the night moaning and groaning. Hopefully the doctors can figure out a way for her to be more comfortable. We think she is affected by the superfortified formula and all of her medicines. The only problem is that sometimes she throws up the medicine five minutes after she takes it.

We cannot wait until both kids are home for good. It should only be a few more days.

172 December 12, 2006

Julia went to the pulmonologist today. She weighs 9 lbs 2.3 oz. The pulmonologist is happy with her growth. She also told us that Julia's lungs sound good, and it is time to start weaning her from the oxygen. She was on .2 liters, and we are going to put her on .1 liters during the day for a few weeks to see how she handles it. If that works, we'll try it twenty-four hours.

Mom sneaked up to see Ronan and even got to give him a bottle. In her unprofessional opinion, he seems psychologically unharmed from his procedure last night. Physically everything is healing as it should be.

173 December 13, 2006

Ronan gained forty grams overnight and weighs just slightly less than eight pounds. He had a final head ultrasound, and it was completely normal with good maturation. This is a huge relief for us. He slept well overnight and had a nice nap this morning. He took his bottle for Dawn with no spit-ups. He is still scheduled to come home tomorrow. Mommy and Daddy will go in the morning to get him. His total hospital stay will be 160 days. If someone had told us he would be there for 160 days on July 8, we never would have made it. It was hard enough for us to hear that he would at least be there until his due date.

He is really doing great. He is alert and active and loves to see what is going on around him. Now the real work begins. We will work with him every day to aid his development. We'll make sure he has lots of tummy time, lots of playing, and storytelling.

Julia had another restless night, but did well on her reduced oxygen yesterday. Today the early intervention social worker paid a visit to do an assessment of her. This agency will help us develop a set of goals for both kids and refer us to any specialists that are required to help. It is important to monitor the kids closely and give them a kick-start if they appear to be struggling in any particular area.

Grandma Gilda will be arriving tomorrow night to help out for a few weeks. Mommy and Daddy will need all the help they can get. The forecast is for temperatures in the upper sixties so Ronan will start out his new life at home with plenty of walks to the park in the next few days. Oh, and he needs to decide what kind of puppy he wants.

Nurse Amy came to stay with Julia this afternoon while Mom and Dad went to the hospital. It was a very busy evening. We reviewed all we had learned about the TPN pump and the feeding pump. Then we gave Ronan a bath. He just leaned back and relaxed. There is a marked change in his demeanor once he hits the water. Next, Mommy got to use her new skills to apply a new sterile dressing on a real baby after Dawn showed her how to restrain Ronan's arms so he couldn't help with the process. Ronan was very well behaved during the procedure, but it is still much easier on the mannequin. Our secret weapon was the pacifier. Ronan is very tolerant of almost anything when he has his paci in his mouth.

One thing Mommy has been struggling with is how to handle Ronan's bris milah. Bris means covenant and milah means to cut. Normally, a mohel performs the circumcision and says prayers to welcome the baby as a Jew. During this ceremony, the baby is also given a Jewish name. We don't currently belong to a synagogue, and the hospital does not have a mohel or a Jewish chaplain on staff. The UNC chaplain did a lot of calling around to the community and came up with a creative solution.

Someone from the Jewish federation provided the prayers, and the chaplain was going to read them for us. However, one of the respiratory therapists who has taken an interest in the twins and has a background in divinity volunteered to do the service. RT Chris printed the prayers off the Internet and read them in Hebrew and in English.

We also had a naming ceremony and gave Ronan the Hebrew name Beryl after my grandfather Bernie. Ronan's middle name is also Bradley after Ed's dad and my grandfather. Since Chris knew Ronan and was comfortable with us, it was a very nice ceremony. Chris also does calligraphy and will write the prayers on parchment for us to keep as a memory of the service. We know it wasn't technically correct, but we thought it was a perfect solution for us.

In the future, we plan to have a naming ceremony for Julia too. We will name her Rahel after her Grandma Ruth. Her English middle name is Rachel after Grandma Ruth.

I got teary too!

December 13, 2006, at 8:04 AM EST

Nicole—don't feel bad about worrying over the circumcision. I got really teary eyed too and had a hard time letting go of Jack to let him get snipped. However, I felt it was in his best interest for many, many reasons (which I won't list here, but I'd be happy to tell you if you wanted) and that helped the sniffles go away. Plus, their memory doesn't really start sticking until months, so you're just fine. I can't think of a single thing I remember before age three, and after that my memory is sketchy at best. Remember, the medicine they give during the procedure is really good, and if he looked comfy afterward then no worries!

Amber

175 December 14, 2006

Ronan is home—for good. Ronan just arrived home a few minutes ago. He is very happy to be home. He is hungry, so Mommy is feeding him his first bottle with his entire family around him. Sister Julia is snoozing and letting the R man have some of the spotlight for a few moments.

160 days later we have both of our children where they belong. We would like to thank everybody who has helped make this day possible. From the folks at Centre OB/GYN, for acting so fast on July 7 to Rex Hospital, to the transport team, to all the wonderful people in the labor and delivery at UNC. Many thanks to all the NICU staff that helped save our babies' lives. We cannot adequately express our gratitude to you all for your efforts and dedication over the past five months.

Specials thanks to Nurses Amy, Dawn, Lauren, Katie, and Linda for managing the kids personally. Many thanks to NNPs Elizabeth, David, and Joanne for always being willing to answer our questions or reassure us. A special thanks to all the doctors, especially Dr. Wood, for putting the plan in place to get our boy home. Also to the surgical staff, Dr. Lange especially, for saving Ronan's life on several occasions and for giving Julia the opportunity to thrive. We have left off a ton of people at the hospitals, but thanks to everyone. And thanks to everybody who took the time to read our blog. This has been a huge help to us mentally. Everyone's notes and thoughts really helped us get through the truly dark days.

And a special thanks to our "rocks." The rocks know who they are, and we appreciate the way they saved us in the early days, the late days, and all the days in between. Thanks again to everyone!

I'm so proud of you, Ronan!

December 14, 2006, at 10:24 AM EST

I am so sad that my little Ronan is leaving me . . . and that I don't get to be there to discharge him, but I am so happy that he can finally go home where he can grow and thrive! He was such a good boy yesterday. No fussing until 7:00 p.m. (of course . . . during shift change). He must have known it was my last day at work with him! I'll come see you all later today or tomorrow.

Lots of love,
Dawn

Woohoo!

December 14, 2006, at 9:47 AM EST

What a day to celebrate! I have longed to see this post . . . every day of your 160! Woohoo!

Aimee

Part 4

Reality Check: The Ride Does Not Ever End, but the Rewards Are Enormous

*** *Things to think about*

- Your child may have medical issues for some time after he is released from the NICU.
- Your child may have developmental delays due to her prematurity.
- Your child may be smaller than other children his age.
- Take advantage of government programs that are available to you.
- Love your child and be patient with her and together you will get through it.
- When your preemie hits a milestone, it is even sweeter than when a full-term baby does.
- It's all worth it in the end because this is your baby.

176 December 15, 2006

Yesterday was a really long day. We spent several hours at the hospital tying up loose ends and speaking to the GI doctors. It was very exciting carrying Ronan out of the hospital for the first time and loading everyone up in the car.

Things were quite hectic when we arrived home. Two are definitely harder than one especially when one needs a lot of medical attention. The nurses from the infusion company arrived shortly after we got home with piles and piles of medical equipment. They brought a pump, syringes, alcohol wipes, tubing, TPN, special vitamins, IV pole, minibackpacks, and the list goes on and on. We couldn't see the kitchen when they were done. They were very friendly and patient, but it was a lot to take in after such a long day.

Between the continuous feedings and the TPN, there are many steps to master. It is very important to keep everything sterile so Ronan does not get an infection in his Broviac. We are desperate to do it right so we don't harm

> our baby, but there is a lot to remember. When we were training, there were no screaming children to interrupt the intense concentration it takes to perform these complicated tasks.
>
> Both kids made it through the night and so did Mommy and Daddy. Ronan was overwhelmed by everything, so it took a long time for him to fall asleep. Many thanks to Nurse Dawn for coming over and helping us get him set up on his IV and making sure he fell asleep. Big thanks to Nurse Amy who also came by to lend her support. Julia was awake for a good chunk of the night, but we suspect it was hard sharing her bed after being alone for so long. Grandma Gilda arrived around 11:00 p.m. last night after a four-hour fog delay at the Philadelphia airport and has already been a huge help to us. We are quite tired, but so happy to have both of the kids home. We can always catch up on sleep later. Right now we just want to enjoy having them with us.

Today I am definitely feeling the pressure. I was all cool at the hospital, thinking I knew what I was in for and was prepared to handle anything. After a very long night with very little sleep, I'm running out of steam. My mom and I tried to pick up the house and get some of the medical clutter organized. There is so much to do with so little time that we will have to work hard to prioritize and organize ourselves. I guess in that respect it is a lot like my paying job. Caring for one child and going to the hospital every other day are starting to seem like a picnic compared to this. I'm trying to remember that I found it very difficult too when we first brought Julia home.

The nurse from the infusion company came by at 8:00 a.m. to help us disconnect the continuous feedings. It is much easier to disconnect than to connect. She came back in the late afternoon to do another review on how to hang the TPN. It turns out that the pediatric pharmacist is concerned about the stability of our TPN setup, and we will have a totally different setup tomorrow involving several new pumps. However, I'm sure some of the steps will remain the same. Next a courier arrived to deliver a whole new package of medical equipment that needs to be refrigerated. Our refrigerator looks like it belongs in a hospital.

The nurse said we could call her when it came time to hang the TPN. I didn't anticipate having to call her. Ed and I went upstairs and laid out all of our equipment. We carefully washed our hands like we've been told and got started. Hooking up the g-tube and continuous feeds went fairly smoothly with few missteps. Between the two of us, we remembered enough to successfully get it started.

The TPN was a different story. In the hospital, all the nurses dislike hanging TPN. They do it at the end of the day shift, and no matter which pod the kids are in or which nurses are on duty, there is always some grumbling. It is definitely not their favorite task.

We both completely blanked in several places and had to call the nurse at home four times to get further direction. She calmly reminded us, "I'm right near the phone and ready to help when you got stuck." We were both getting pretty frustrated and starting to snap at each other. It didn't help that Julia and Ronan were both crying during the exercise. Eventually with the nurse's help, we finally got it running. I'm sure it will get easier, but right now it seems pretty complicated. I'm sure being tired and having big headaches did not help the situation.

Another thing that had me feeling frustrated and like a bad mother was Ronan's feedings. He is supposed to get continuous feeds from 8:00 p.m. to 8:00 a.m. and to be bottle-fed four times from 8:00 a.m. to 8:00 p.m. I got a little backed up, and one of his feeds was an hour late. I didn't feel comfortable giving him his fourth feed right before he went on the continuous feeds as this could cause him to spit up. The nurse was gracious about it, but she said we really need to be careful and suggested that I try to space out the feeds every 2 to 2 ½ hours tomorrow to make sure he gets four and possibly five. She also suggested I weigh him tomorrow morning so we can make sure he is not losing weight due to the missed feed. We don't want the GI doctor to think she made a mistake by sending him home too early.

It will get easier.
It will get easier.
It will get easier.
It will get easier.

There is nothing like the power of a short mantra. Wish us all good luck tonight!

There were some neat moments today. For right now, we have both kids in a crib in our room. It is so wonderful to see them together. The first day they really didn't pay any attention to each other. Tonight they seem to be noticing each other a little more when they are in the crib together. My mom, Ed, and I all stood around the crib watching them. We turned on the mobile, and both kids appeared to be watching it. We knew Ronan loved his mobile, but Julia seems to have an interest in it too.

Julia seems to be maturing. She was in great spirits and behaved so well all day. It's almost like she is giving us a break because she knows Ronan needs a little extra attention right now. She is also starting to sleep better at night despite Ronan's late night escapades. We're enjoying watching her pass into the next stage.

Grandma Gilda is really enjoying her time here with the kids. She loves to talk to them and play with them. She is also a huge help around the house with cleaning, organizing, cooking, and doing bottle duty. We'd like her to stay until they go to kindergarten. Grandpa Michael probably wouldn't be too happy about that.

177 December 18, 2006

Just a quick note. We feel very lucky to have Ronan home with us, but now we know why the nurses don't like hanging TPN. It is very tedious, and there are a couple of steps that always give us trouble.

Ronan went in to see the GI doctor today. He weighs 8 lbs 5.5 oz. She had a lot of questions about Ronan's habits but didn't have any changes for us today. They will continue to monitor him closely. He doesn't have to go back until early January.

Julia has been very well behaved since Ronan arrived. She seems to understand that Mommy and Daddy are a little stressed by Ronan's medical needs. Julia has become much more aware of her surroundings, and rumor has it that she is even starting to smile. She is sleeping very well at night despite Ronan's best attempts to keep her up.

Ronan and Julia are enjoying their first Hanukah. Every night after we light the candles we darken the room so they can enjoy the lights. Tonight is the fourth night.

178 December 19, 2006

We have become a bit frustrated with the TPN process. We thought we had the process down well, but then things started to change. We have received conflicting directions on proper procedures, unfamiliar supplies, problems with the pumps, and not a lot of support. Once again Nurses Amy and Dawn have been a huge help in getting us through this. We are not quite sure who should be coordinating this, but it doesn't seem to be going smoothly.

While we are very happy to have Ronan home, 8:00 p.m. has become a stressful and nerve-wracking time. Every night it is a battle to get his continuous feeds and TPN up and running. Each night we encounter a different problem. Today we needed more Y-adapters because they only sent a few. Nicole called at 8:00 a.m. and again at 6:30 p.m. to get information about when the supplies were arriving. The courier finally arrived at 7:30 p.m. The Y-adapters we received are not the same as the ones we used in training, but nobody warned us of this before they arrived. There was also some confusion about whether we needed to flush Ronan's g-tube after feeds.

On the lighter side, both kids went to the doctor today. Ronan weighs 8 lbs 8 oz give or take a few ounces. Julia weighs 9 lbs 12 oz. The doctor was impressed with both kids and their progress. Nurses Dawn and Amy stopped by today for a visit. Dawn helped give Ronan a bath.

179 December 21, 2006

Last night went a bit better. A visiting nurse came and reviewed each procedure with us in detail. All we need is some help from time to time, but we were told there are not enough pediatric nurses in the area to provide this type of support. The nurse was very nice and extremely helpful. Unfortunately, the lipid pump clogged at 4:00 a.m., so we still need to get that resolved. We have also come to the conclusion that we are on our own with this. We need to learn to do it and learn to handle the stress that comes with it. Ronan is seeing the surgeon today about his hernia. He also has an eye exam and possibly a visit with the GI doctor if there is time. Tomorrow he visits the speech therapist. He is a busy boy these days, and so is Mommy.

181 December 21, 2006

The good news is that Ronan's eyes are mature. He is a little farsighted which is normal in term babies, but unusual in preemies. He does have a membrane that was supposed to go away called persistent pupillary membrane. It won't affect his sight, and the doctor is not concerned with it.

Dr. Kirk Gelatt tells us that persistent pupillary membrane (PPM) is a condition of the eye involving remnants of a fetal membrane that persist as strands of tissue crossing the pupil. The pupillary membrane in mammals exists in the fetus as a source of blood supply for the lens. It normally atrophies from the time of birth to the age of four to eight weeks. PPM occurs when this atrophy is incomplete. It generally does not cause any symptoms. The strands can connect to the cornea or lens but most commonly to other parts of the iris. Attachment to the cornea can cause small corneal opacities while attachment to the lens can cause small cataracts. Using topical atropine to dilate the pupil may help break down PPMs.

Our TPN problems continue. Now we have a setup with a pump for the lipids and a pump for the TPN itself. The first few nights, we had a three-in-one bag that included TPN and lipids and ran through one pump.

We are still having problems with the lipid pump alarming at night. The alarm indicates there is a "lower occlusion." We've heard all sorts of theories about why this might be happening, but they seem to be taking a long time to present a solution.

The pediatric surgery nurse practitioner looked at Ronan's Broviac today and made some suggestions. She said that we were not flushing it with enough saline and heparin. She increased the amounts on these and that may help prevent the occlusions. She also thought that Ronan might have some fibers that were narrowing the passages of the Broviac, so she gave him a medicine called TPA through his Broviac. TPA or tissue plasminogen activator is a thrombolytic agent (clot-busting drug). We'll see tonight whether any of these changes helped. I'm very encouraged by the TPA theory.

The other change they are going to make is to implement a brand-new TPN system. As I understand it, we are going back to one bag and one pump. The one bag will have a chamber separating the TPN and lipids, and we'll break it before starting the line. A nurse will be coming tomorrow to show us what to do.

We were told today that Ronan has a pretty severe hernia on the right side and a minor one on the left side. This is extremely common in preemies. Unfortunately, we are in a tough position with this situation. Normally they don't like to do surgery on a hernia while the infant is on TPN since TPN affects liver function. They would prefer to do surgery on the infant three months after he stops the TPN. If they do it earlier, the problem could return. If he stops TPN in three to eight months, it could be almost a year before they do the surgery. The downside of waiting is that the hernia could strangulate his bowels. This could put him in danger of losing more of his bowels. He really can't afford to lose more of his bowels right now. In addition, if the bowel strangulates it could cause him a huge amount of pain.

We're leaning toward doing it sooner rather than later, but the surgeon who did Ronan's other surgeries is not available to even look at it until January 8. We were hoping to see her today.

I'm not sure what is going on with Julia since I spent five and a half hours at the hospital today. I know they are busy, but I really think that is a little much.

Thanks, Grandma Gilda, for all your help. There is no way we would have been able to manage this week without you.

We've all been enjoying the twins' first Hanukah. Every night we bring everyone into the kitchen, light the candles, and sing the Hanukah song. We turn off all the lights so the kids can focus on the candles. Next year at this time, they'll be fighting over who gets to pick the candle colors each night.

182 December 26, 2006

Everybody had a great weekend and holiday. We think we finally have Ronan's TPN problems resolved. The pharmacist suggested a dual chamber IV bag which has worked great so far. The best part is that we only have to hook it to one pump instead of the two pumps we were using before. Ronan sleeps through the night. We do change him at least once each night since his nickname is "poopy pants." Everybody who visits after not seeing him for a few days says he is getting bigger.

Julia is also doing well. She is all smiles these days. This morning she smiled and cooed at Daddy before he left for work. Yesterday Grandpa arrived, so it was nice having everybody together. We've taken a lot of pictures, so keep a lookout for updates. As the year draws to a close, we reflect on what has happened so far. The year started off with the exciting news of the pregnancy, sank with the twins' premature arrival, but is back on top again. We are so thankful to have both kids home. Yes, they scream, and yes, we are tired; but then we are well aware of how things could have turned out. We realize that we are truly lucky. Happy Holidays to everyone.

183 December 26, 2006

Not an hour after the visiting nurse left, Daddy arrived home from work to find a rather lethargic blue Ronan. We hooked up the pulsox to check his oxygen saturation rates and heart rate. The oxygen saturation rate was bouncing around, and the heart rate was twice as fast as it normally is for Ronan. Oddly enough, we have two pulsox units so we tested Ronan on both. Very similar numbers came up on the second one.

We took his temperature, and it was very high, so we quickly called the pediatrician's office. The pediatrician has night hours for emergencies and told us to come in right away. The doctor took one look at him and rushed us down to the emergency room. She said something to the receptionist, and Ronan was in an emergency bed quicker than we could comprehend.

In the emergency room, they gave Ronan oxygen, IV fluids, and Tylenol. He bounced back quickly, but obviously they needed to find out what caused these problems. This hospital does not handle complicated cases with ex-preemies, so they prepared to send us back to UNC. The pediatrician later told us that when she heard it was Ronan coming in, she knew it was not going to be a quick case. She let her office staff go home but stayed with us for several hours to make sure everything was OK. She was awfully kind. It still amazes us how much everyone cares.

Needless to say, we were not thrilled about sending Ronan back to the hospital. Germ wise, a hospital is one of the worst places we can be, especially during cold and flu season. Unfortunately, at this point, we did not have a choice. They took him by ambulance to UNC, admitted him, and did some tests which all came back normal. After a long night, Ronan was assigned a room, and all finally got to sleep around 3:00 a.m.

184 December 27, 2006

In order to rule out an infection, blood cultures need to grow for forty-eight hours. Nothing has appeared as of yet, and if the cultures are clean on Friday, he will be able to go home. In anticipation of a possible infection, they put him on very strong antibiotics. If they waited until the forty-eight hours were over, it could be too late.

Mommy and Daddy came home for a couple of hours to shower and see Julia, but we will be back at the hospital tonight. Just when we think the worst is behind us, fate gives us a punch in the gut. We will post an update tomorrow.

185 December 28, 2006

Ronan is doing better today. "Gram negative rods" showed up in his culture. This is a very general identification and is usually associated with an intestinal infection. They will need some more time for the cultures to grow before they can identify it more specifically.

Ronan is scheduled to have his hernia repaired on January 5. His regular surgeon agreed that in Ronan's case, it was better to do the surgery sooner rather than later. Hopefully we can get this problem repaired along with the infection. Today he was in good spirits and was even smiling at the nurses and Mommy and Daddy. He is such a good boy. All he wants is to be held occasionally and his pacifier. We are rather disappointed with how the different medical teams fail to communicate. It seems they expect the parents to get all sides talking to each other.

Ronan has a tentative release date of Sunday or Monday.

186 December 29, 2006

Mommy spent the night with Ronan, and Daddy will stay home tonight. Grandma and Grandpa are leaving tomorrow. They have been a huge help with Julia. Julia has also been a huge help. She is now sleeping through the night and is usually in good spirits during the day.

Now if we can only help the boy recover, perhaps some of this incredible stress can be reduced. Good riddance to 2006. May 2007 be a much better year for us all.

187 December 29, 2006

The cultures came back this afternoon, and Ronan's infection was identified as E. coli. The doctor was able to take him off the extra strong antibiotics and put him on one that specifically targets this infection. We hope he can come home in a couple of days.

That Ronan never gets a break!

December 29, 2006, at 8:32 PM EST

With luck, this will be his last infection . . . better to get it all over with in 2006 so he can start 2007 on an upswing. He's so talented at catching all those little germies . . . but trust me that he is getting stronger and more resistant all the time which will do him good as he gets older. My heart goes out to all of you, and with luck, you'll all be back home together really soon! Good girl, Julia, for being patient with Mom and Dad and Ronan while this is going on . . . you'll get your brother back before you know it!

Amber

Wow! E. coli! Whoa!

December 29, 2006, at 07:23 PM EST

How in the world does that even happen with a baby? Yuck, yuck, yuck! I'm so sorry you are dealing with that but grateful they know and can fix it.
Hang in there, Ronan!
Way to catch that change, Mom and Dad. You have most certainly saved his life once again!

Aimee

188 December 30, 2006

Much to Julia's disappointment, Grandma and Grandpa left this morning. We will really miss having them around. Mom and Dad are getting used to the routine of swapping places every twenty-four hours. Today Daddy is at home with Julia, and Mom is at the hospital with Ronan.

Ronan seems to be feeling OK. He is on a ten-day course of antibiotics for the E. coli infection. They are leaning on keeping him until next Saturday or Sunday. He has to at least stay until his blood cultures come back negative for the virus on either Sunday or Monday. They also have to make sure the antibiotics are working properly. I asked the GI doctor about the possibility of letting him come home for a few days before his surgery. She has some objections to this but promised she would consider it.

Ronan has had several visitors from the NICU. His primary night nurse, Katie, came to visit the other day, and Nurse Amy came by to say hello. Today NNP Elizabeth came to visit. She was surprised at how big he has gotten. Nurse Dawn is out of town, so she has not been able to visit, but Ronan knows she is thinking about him.

189 December 31, 2006

Ronan is doing much better today. His blood tests came back negative which means the antibiotics are working. He is holding up well being in the hospital again. Mommy and Daddy, however, are not doing as well. It is very difficult being apart all the time as one of us must be with Ronan at the hospital. There is no downtime these days. We are either with Ronan at the hospital or with Julia at home. The only break is driving between the hospital and home. We hope we will be able to handle it for the rest of the week and then have our boy back home again.

190 January 1, 2007

It was a quiet new year. Daddy stayed with Ronan overnight. He was a good boy and is eating well. He is alert and happy.

Julia is also doing very well. Daddy stayed with her today while Mommy went and stayed with Ronan. Ronan is still scheduled to have his surgery on Friday. We hope he can come home next weekend.

191 January 2, 2007

Ronan weighed in at 9 lbs 8 oz today. He has gained a half pound since being in the hospital. His blood tests continue to come back negative. Today his surgeon, Dr. Lange, came by to talk about his hernia surgery on Friday. As we talked about it, Ronan started to cry. I guess he knew what we were talking about. Dr. Lange says he should be able to leave Saturday or Sunday. We cannot wait.

Julia has passed the ten-pound mark. She went to get her RSV shot today and as usual was a real trouper. Tonight is Daddy's turn at the hospital on the pullout couch.

192 January 4, 2007

Ronan is going under the knife tomorrow. The anesthesiologist came by with some general questions. She told us he will be going to surgery around noon time. Please think good thoughts for Ronan tomorrow as he completes what we hope will be his last surgery. He was in a very good mood today. He was smiling at Mommy and Daddy and flirting like crazy with all the nurses.

Julia continues to be a wonderful baby. She is very cheerful and loves to smile and is now starting to verbalize a bit.

193 January 5, 2007

Ronan went down to surgery about 1:30 p.m. We went and stayed with him until they came to get him. As usual he was very interested in what was going on around him. His surgeon said it should take about an hour and a half unless they have to do both sides. Hernia surgery is very common for preemies, but as we know every time they operate, they are taking a chance. The plan is to discharge him tomorrow afternoon if everything goes as planned. We will post an update when he is back from surgery.

194 January 5, 2007

Ronan is back from surgery and did fine. Only one side needed repair. He is a bit cranky but has been given drugs to help him with the pain. He is scheduled to come home tomorrow.

195 January 7, 2007

After much negotiation on Saturday, Mom was able to spring Ronan from the joint. He enjoyed a light nap on the way home and was immediately whisked into the double stroller for a walk with the family. He received warm greetings from all the neighbors. His first night home was uneventful, and the whole family enjoyed a leisurely morning together.

196 January 10, 2007

Ronan is settling in quite nicely at home again. We think he is interested in his sister. He will watch her intently and, when he has the chance, snuggles up with her.

Mina Peggy arrived this afternoon for a visit. She hasn't seen the kids since the first week back in July when they weighed two pounds or less. She was very impressed. Both kids love snuggling with Mina and look forward to a nice visit and walks with her on the warm days. Mommy is doing quite well with the two kids. It is a long day for Mommy and Daddy, but it is what we have been hoping for since July. We promise to take some new pictures soon. The time never seems to be there, but this week we will make the effort.

Look at those bright eyes!

January 13, 2007, at 08:26 PM EST

Oh, you guys . . . your kids look so great! I can't tell you how happy it makes me to see them together at home with their eyes open and taking in everything! Julia has gorgeous features (and those fantastic eyes), and Ronan is just as handsome and laid-back as he's always been . . . what a trouper. They've come so far since I first met them in July, and I'm so happy that they're both home and getting into a routine (which will change all the time, so don't get used to anything). We think of you, guys, all the time, and when we're all over this terrible cold at my house, we'll be sure to come over for a nice walk!

Amber

197 January 14, 2007

The kids are really enjoying their visit with Mina Peggy. Mina Peggy is really enjoying her visit with the kids. She is rarely seen without at least one of them in her arms. We've taken several family walks during the warm weather, and Mina has been a huge help with feedings and diaper changes.

Julia is still on oxygen although we have started weaning her to lower levels. We removed her cannula for the pictures. She went to the Special Infant Care Clinic on Thursday and weighs 10 lbs 9.3 oz. The doctors are very pleased with her development. Ronan's Special Infant Care Clinic is scheduled for early February.

Ronan's bilirubin levels are lower again. It is really reflecting in his color. He is still kind of fussy but seems to be settling into life at home. It took several weeks for Julia to feel comfortable, and we need to be patient with Ronan since he's been through so much more. He has made a lot of progress in the week he has been home from the hospital, but we still need to work with him more on his feeding and tummy time.

It is so wonderful to have everyone at home.

198 January 16, 2007

Just a quick note about our latest setback. We hope it is a minor one. Ronan was looking a little peculiar this morning, and he had a temperature. With any normal baby, we'd just give him some Tylenol and watch him. With a baby that has a central line, we can't take chances like that. We've seen before how quickly Ronan can take a turn for the worse. After six hours in the emergency room, we were transferred to a room on the seventh floor at UNC Hospitals. They've ruled out the flu and RSV, and they drew blood cultures to check for infections. If nothing grows in the cultures, the best-case scenario is that we could spring him as early as Thursday afternoon.

Ronan seemed fine, and his temperature was back to normal when it was taken twice in the ER. He even managed to smile for the nurses and make himself adorable as usual. It would be easy to say we are disappointed and upset, but at this time, we are pretty drained of the ability to think these things. Once again we will be taking turns between home and the hospital.

Julia and Mina spent a quiet day at home. Mina is leaving tomorrow morning. Thanks for all the help! We're sorry to end her visit this way.

200 January 18, 2007

Ronan may be able to come home this afternoon. His cultures have been clean as we near the forty-eight-hour mark. The doctors are very pleased with his progress. They've also increased his feedings so they can start to decrease his TPN volumes. Once the TPN is discontinued, they normally like to wait a few weeks before they remove the central line because they need to make sure he can continue to gain weight without the assistance of the TPN. We're hoping that since he has gained several pounds since he started the TPN, his intestines are more capable of absorbing all the nutrients he needs. However, we're getting ahead of ourselves. It will be some time before we are able to get him totally off the TPN.

Daddy stayed over last night at the hospital and is waiting for the word that Ronan can leave. Ronan is in good spirits but insists on being held constantly.

201 January 18, 2007

Ronan came home this afternoon—that's really good news. Unfortunately Mommy has caught a stomach bug, so she is confined to her room. Daddy will now have three people to take care of after two long days at the hospital. Thanks to Amber for going to pick up Ronan and Daddy and special thanks to our neighbor Nancy who watched Julia this afternoon while Nicole was sick. We owe them, big time.

A stomach bug does not even begin to describe the day I had. I woke up in the morning kind of excited that I had "Julia-at-home" duty instead of "Ronan-at-hospital" duty. I was also excited about the possibility of Ronan's being discharged from the hospital. I fed Julia around 8:30 a.m. and took a shower. My stomach was bothering me a little, but I didn't think too much of it. I called to see how Ronan was, and Ed told me that he had had a good night and everything was in place to discharge him as long as the cultures were still clean at the forty-eight-hour mark.

Oddly enough it had snowed the night before—rare in North Carolina. It was less than an inch but enough to gum up the works. Schools were closed, and many parents were forced to take the day off from work. My teacher-friend Lori called to see how we were doing and to say hello. I had a nice chat with her, but after that, things started to take a turn for the worse.

I had Julia in bed with me sitting on her Boppy. She really likes her Boppy and is usually content to spend at least an hour sitting in it looking around and chattering. My stomach hurt so much that I grabbed the garbage can from the bathroom and placed it by the bed. There was a famous incident in 1994 that taught me that vomit stains do not come out of carpeting. Getting to the bathroom was a little bit of a problem as I was feeling kind of dizzy and worn out. I also was feeling pretty feverish with alternating chills and sweats.

At that point, I stopped to consider my options. I did not want Julia to get sick, plus my ability to take care of her was going downhill quickly. Ed needed to be at the hospital with Ronan. Our parents were very far away. Lori said she had to go into school to work on her grades plus her husband was sick, so it was apparent she could not assist. I left a message for my other teacher-friend, but it turned out he had gotten to school before it was cancelled and just stayed there. As I muddled through my options, I felt the urge to throw up. I won't go into details except to say I was on the floor on all fours with my head in the garbage can wanting to die.

Now would be a good time to put an emergency plan into action (if we had had one). I made an executive decision to call my neighbor Nancy across the street. I don't know her too well, but she is very nice and has taken a huge interest in the kids. In addition, she works part-time from home. In between rounds with the garbage can, I used my laptop to look up her phone number and call her. Miraculously, she was home and willing to come over. She had her daughter home with her because of the snow day.

Fifteen minutes later, I heard the glorious sound of the doorbell. I managed to tote Julia and her oxygen line downstairs and show Nancy where everything was. At that point I honestly believed if I could sleep a few hours, I could come down and relieve her. I went back upstairs again to lie down. It was the most bizarre day. I wasn't sleeping, but I wasn't really awake either. I could not move. This is unusual for me. I never sit still. And Ed wonders where Julia got her energy from? I managed to move a few times to hang out with the garbage can, but it wasn't the kind of experience that made me feel better. It just made me feel worse.

Now, I was dehydrated but afraid to drink any water. I had a huge headache and a high fever, but I was afraid to take an aspirin. It took me a good three hours to drag myself out of bed in search of the aspirin and to finally consume it along with some water.

It was weird. I heard bits and pieces of what was going on downstairs, but it seemed so far away. The hours passed so slowly. I called my husband to tell him I was dying. Ronan was still going to be discharged, and he needed a way home. I called Nurse Amy, but she had plans. I debated with myself and called my friend Amber. I felt bad asking her to go to the hospital on a snow day, during rush hour when she has her own child to take care of, but there was no way I could drive there to pick them up. Fortunately, she was home and willing to do me the favor.

I kept thinking I should go downstairs to relieve my neighbor, but it was beyond my current abilities. Ed arrived home about six, and I heard him thanking everyone profusely. After that, everything started to get a little crazy. It seems like everyone always wants to eat at the same time and the TPN needed to be hung. There was nothing I could do to help. Ed was getting a little stressed after being stuck in a small hospital room with Ronan crying for hours on end. Unfortunately, he was continuing his crying spell at home.

We felt it was important not to expose the kids to me any more than we had. This meant a day home from work for Ed and two children (and an adult) to take care of on his own. After three straight days with no break, he was on edge. Once again, there was nothing I could do to help. He had a really tough Thursday night, Friday, and Saturday morning. Saturday afternoon I washed my hands very thoroughly and rolled up my sleeves to help. What an awful week, starting with Tuesday's hospital admission! At this point, we were both pretty blue. It was great to have Ronan home from the hospital, but caring for two special-needs infants is a huge challenge under the best of circumstances.

The whole week stretched before me. Ed got to go back to work on Monday. I didn't even have that to look forward to. The weather was supposed to be in the forties all week, so there would be no walks. How was I going to entertain these two children all week in the same room? Monday was very gray and cold and depressing. I just could not think a good thought even when Julia smiled her sweet smile at me. Ronan spent much of the day crying in between eating and a few five-minute naps.

I called an old friend and tried to talk it out. She helped me feel a little better. Nurse Amy came over around 4:30 p.m. and took one look at me and said I should go out. Trying not to act too excited, I grabbed my book and got in the car. I ended up at Dairy Queen and bought an ice cream. I got home an hour later, and Ronan was napping and Amy was playing with Julia. Apparently, Ronan was a perfect gentleman the entire time I was gone.

That all changed when I arrived. He woke up and started crying again. I took him for a walk around the downstairs and showed him the baby in the mirror.

Why oh why does he cry so much? Eventually it was time to give him his bottle, which is always a peaceful time. The bottle goes in, and the crying stops.

In the morning, I went into the nursery to disconnect Ronan from his maze of tubes. We moved them into their own room last week. It is so wonderful to have our bedroom back. The kids were lying right next to each other and looked awfully cute. Ronan was flailing his arms and whining and whacking Julia. Julia cried for a minute but quickly stopped. She looked up at me with her bright blue eyes and gave me a big smile. She is such a happy child. If we keep talking to her, we can usually get a couple of smiles in a row. Each smile is accompanied by a mouthful of saliva. She has two teeth coming in in her upper row, and her bibs are soaked in minutes. We're going to have to get out the teething rings soon. Ronan also has two teeth coming in his lower row, but his saliva is still mostly under control. They tell me that with preemies some things develop by their actual age which is six months, and other things develop by their adjusted age which is three months. Teeth fall into the prior category.

Every Tuesday morning the home health care nurse will come by to take Ronan's blood, assess him, and change his Broviac dressing. She is very friendly and easy to get along with, and I really look forward to her visits. She always comes in with a whirlwind of stories and advice. While she worked with Ronan, I wiped Julia down and changed her outfit. The nurse also fed Ronan and gave him a bath. She genuinely seems to enjoy spending time with him. She had a whole list of ideas of things I could do to jazz things up in our lives. She suggested I take the kids to a movie or a bookstore during the day when the weather was cold. She waved away my worries of exposing them to germs. Her recommendation was to keep them covered with a blanket when I needed to and to find a quiet corner somewhere. That is not hard in a movie theater during the day.

After the nurse left, Julia spent a lot of the early afternoon sleeping, so I worked with Ronan. I talked to him, did his stretches to keep him flexible, and practiced having him sit up for head control. He had a few calm moments and even managed a few smiles. Before I knew it, it was time to take him to his GI appointment.

He weighs 10 lbs 12 oz, and the doctor is very happy with his growth and his labs. She also thought his color and tongue were doing a lot better too. For the first time since we started measuring it, his total bilirubin is down to 1.2 which is right at the top of the acceptable range. The rest of his labs looked good too. The great news is that the doctor was so happy with his progress that she agreed to lower his TPN fluid volume by 10 percent. This is the first time we've been able to lower it. I asked the doctor to venture a guess on how long he'd be on it, and she gave me the standard answer, "Everyone is different, it is up to him."

In addition to lowering the TPN fluid volume, we've been increasing his nightly g-tube feedings by 1 ml per hour per week. We've also tried to increase the volume he takes by mouth during the day. The doctor is not concerned by the vomiting he has been doing during some of his bottle-feeds. She said that is normal and sometimes even gets a little worse as the babies become more active. She thinks the mucous in his vomit might have something to do with his tongue thrusts.

I also had a long conversation with the nutritionist. She explained that the formula Ronan is on is good for preemies because the proteins are broken down and it is much easier to digest than other formulas. She is very happy with his weight gain. I asked how we would wean him off continuous feeds. She explained that we'd have to wean him completely off the TPN before we started weaning him off the continuous feedings. She did not want to guess at how long it would take to get him off the continuous feedings, but she did warn me that he would have to go through a major illness and six months of no g-tube feeds before they would remove the g-tube.

They want to avoid putting him through another surgery in case he needs the g-tube again. Kids who go through a g-tube surgery tend to lose a lot of weight and sometimes have trouble gaining again. Six months gives them time to make sure that he can gain weight without it and gives the doctors the comfort level to remove it. After he is off the TPN, they will slowly cut the number of hours per night that he is on continuous feeds and make sure he can tolerate extra bottle-feeds during the day.

Ed talked to his manager today about taking a six-week leave when I go back to work at the end of March. She seemed to be OK with the idea of it but reminded Ed that she doesn't have any choice. The Family Medical Leave Act (FMLA) is a federal law that allows workers to take up to twelve weeks of unpaid leave a year to care for a newborn or ill family member. Since they were so generous to Ed with time off when the kids were born, he promised he will be flexible with them during his unpaid leave. I think it is really important for him (or any parent) to spend some time bonding with the babies while they are young. I'm not crazy about imposing new laws on employers, but it is a shame that this country does not follow the lead of other countries that give generous paid or unpaid leave to both parents after the birth of a child. I suppose we should be happy with FMLA. It's more than parents in the United States had twenty years ago. However, it is still not flexible or realistic enough.

Great gains, Ronan!

January 25, 2007, at 12:52 PM EST

Wow! I checked on the last posts, and do you realize that last week Julia weighed in at 10 lbs 9 oz and now (just one week later) Ronan has matched and beaten her weigh-in? That's fantastic weight gain by Ronan (and you know Julia isn't doing bad, either) . . . see . . . just getting them home makes them grow like weeds! We used to gauge Jack's weight by the weight of other kitchen products so now you have two sacks of potatoes (or flour if you prefer). Of course, potatoes and flour sacks aren't quite so wiggly.

Amber

January 26, 2007

Ronan has been having some issues with reflux. After eating, he starts this horrendous coughing which may or may not result in a spit-up. Some of the large spit-ups can be close to an entire feeding's worth of milk. He looks so uncomfortable; I'm surprised he doesn't refuse to eat. We've tried adjusting his reflux medications, but he still is very uncomfortable. He also has a lot of extra mucous in his throat which makes things worse for him. We really hate seeing him so uncomfortable. Julia did a lot of spitting up when she got home, but she has mostly outgrown it. She does still have some reflux and arches her body when she feels uncomfortable. We hope that Ronan will soon outgrow his feeding problems too.

Last night Julia ate at 8:30 p.m. and did not wake up until 6:00 a.m. She is really getting to be a big girl. Ed called me in when he went to feed her. "You've got to see this," he called. When they went to bed, he placed them in their crib about six inches apart, both heads at the top. When he went to feed her, she was upside down—her feet to his head and she had him trapped in the corner. They both looked pretty comfortable, though. I think having his sister close really makes him feel better.

It's been very cold this week, and we haven't been able to get out as much, so Mom decided it was time for a field trip. We went to the drive-through pharmacy and the drive-through credit union and then headed to our friend Aimee's new photography studio to say hello. She took pictures of the kids when they were in the NICU and will be doing another session with them in a few weeks. Aimee had her twin girls with her at work, and they were fascinated with the kids, especially with Ronan. Ronan and Julia really seemed to appreciate the change of scenery. Maybe they get bored being cooped up in the house. I know that I do. It's exciting to see someone follow their dream. We all hope that Aimee's business grows by leaps and bounds.

I think the hardest part of raising young special-needs twins is the sheer volume of work. Between making formula, changing diapers, wiping down babies, feeding them, managing medications, talking to insurance companies and doctors, washing clothes, soothing tempers, and playing with them, a day can go by fast. Playing with them is the fun part, though. Unfortunately, that doesn't always get on the top of the list. Neither does picking up around the house. Sigh!

January 27, 2007

Both kids are starting to make some developmental progress. Julia is learning how to use her voice. Sometimes she seems surprised at some of the noises when they come out of her mouth. She is also developing her muscles by kicking and shaking her fists. She has started to show some interest in her toys. We've even seen her grab them. Last night she was watching her brother intently with a big smile.

Ronan is also starting to make some developmental strides. He is starting to show some interest in toys, especially his new stuffed octopus. He can grab it and hold it. This morning he was batting at a blue elephant that is hanging from his swing. He also has started to smile in the mornings. He is very happy when he first wakes up. He has some more work to do on building up the muscles in his neck during tummy time. His tongue issues seem to be improving, but he has terrible reflux problems. He loves to cover Mom and Dad with secondhand milk, thus creating a lot of adult laundry to go along with all of the baby laundry. His overall disposition seems to be improving, and it is nice to see him settling into his new life.

January 28, 2007

Our friends Colt and Catherine offered to come over and watch Ronan and Julia for a few hours today so Mommy and Daddy could get out of the house and do something together. We went to brunch at a nice restaurant and did a little shopping. It was wonderful to get out of the house and spend some time alone. Amazingly, both kids were perfectly behaved the whole time we were gone, and Colt and Catherine offered to come back again another time. Ronan really seemed to take a liking to Colt.

January 31, 2007

Yesterday Ronan went to the hospital for his swallow study. They put him on an x-ray machine and fed him thin barium and thick barium and took x-rays of the liquid going down his throat. It looked like it was catching at one point and taking a while to go all the way down. The speech therapist said she would look at the film overnight, and we could review her findings in the morning.

I've got a bad cold, and I am worried about passing it on to the kids. Unfortunately, I am the primary caregiver right now, and it is hard for me to cut off contact with them. I'm trying to wash my hands as frequently as possible, but it's hard when I am sneezing all the time. I'm so tired that it is hard to keep going.

I felt pretty lousy this morning when I woke up, so I asked Ed to take Ronan to the speech therapist this morning. He is frustrated because all of these doctors' appointments take away from his time at work. I understand that, but we don't have family around, and sometimes we have to make sacrifices.

We've looked into getting part-time private nursing care to ease some of the medical burden, but there seems to be a shortage of pediatric nurses in the area. We've also discussed getting a mother's helper or babysitter to come in a few hours a day. People keep telling us that one healthy kid or two healthy twins are overwhelming to care for and that caring for two medically fragile infants is a nearly impossible task even for the most competent caregiver. It takes so much energy to feed them and clean up after them; there is not enough energy left to give them the kind of stimulation they need to catch up developmentally. I try to read to them, talk to them, sing to them, and play with them; but those enrichment activities are hard to keep up for long periods of time because they are constantly interrupted by new requests for feedings. I try to take my cues from the people who come over. I watch everyone interact with the babies and try to get ideas from them.

January 31, 2007

The speech therapist is concerned about Ronan's swallowing. There is a spot where the formula catches and pools due to his poor suck, swallow, and breathing routine. There is a chance that if he breathes while it is pooling it could get sucked into his airway. Further down there is a second spot where the formula is catching as well. For that reason, it looks like rice cereal is out for now. We'll be taking him to the speech therapist frequently to work on these issues. Unfortunately, during his session with the speech therapist, he spit up his entire bottle on Daddy. Despite having a tough time keeping his formula down, he still manages to smile from time to time.

Julia is becoming very vocal. She loves to try out new sounds at all hours of the day and night. Mommy and Daddy are looking for some help to come in a few times a week. All of the appointments, feedings, medicines, and phone calls are beginning to take their toll.

Next week we are going to visit a special pediatric day treatment center for kids with medical needs. There is a chance Ronan can start there shortly and then Julia when there is another spot open. Unlike other daycares, this place is only open to "medically fragile" kids who require special services. The staff includes nurses and physical, speech, occupational, and respiratory therapists that can all help get the twins up to speed with their peers more quickly.

Many years ago, we were driving down a road in Florida. There was one lane each way with water on each side. Every 100 feet or so, there was a yellow sign in the shape of a flag. Each one had one word on it. Patience... Pays... Only... Three... Miles... Until... Passing. I think that is a good motto for life. Unfortunately, being patient is easier said than done. I try to think about it every once in a while when I'm frustrated with something like I am now. I also like the motto This Too Shall Pass. It will, and I'll wish they were infants again. I know time passes quickly, and I'm supposed to enjoy things as they come rather than wishing for the next stage. I also know that we are lucky to have gotten to this stage. Not all preemies do.

208 February 1, 2007

Everybody was home today because of the snow. Unbelievably, it does snow in North Carolina on occasion. Ronan was his usual smiley self in the morning. There was one unfortunate incident when he threw up on his sister and on Ollie the Octopus. Both cleaned up fairly easily.

Julia enjoyed her day, including her time with the activity center and all her stuffed toys. Her favorite seems to be Sam the Seahorse, a gift to Ronan from Nurse Dawn. Overall, it was a quiet day even with Daddy working upstairs and taking some breaks to sneak in a kiss and hug. Tomorrow the kids have appointments to get their RSV shots. Daddy will be going along since Mommy hasn't gotten the swing of transporting two kids at once. We are also going to have the doctor check Ronan's bum since his diaper rash is not getting any better.

209 February 2, 2007

Both kids went to the pediatrician this morning. Daddy came along to help transport and amuse them. Amazingly enough, Ronan has surpassed his sister in the weight department. He weighs 11 lbs 6.5 oz, and Julia weighs 11 lbs 1.5 oz. The doctor was pleased with both weights. She told us that Ronan's weight is "catch-up weight." She said Julia's lungs sound very good. We hope it won't be too much longer with the oxygen. Both kids also got their monthly RSV shot. There was some crying, but fortunately they have short memories. Daddy called Julia a wet noodle after her shot. She was sitting in Mommy's arms slumped over and looking sad.

Next week will be calmer with only a few doctors' appointments and the tour of the daycare center.

February 5, 2007

We had a nice start to the week. Amie from the NICU came over for lunch and a play date with her son, Samuel, who is six months old. He was very interested in the twins. He kept looking back and forth as if he was surprised that there were two of them. He shared his toys; including a very musical hammer that fascinated both kids.

Amie introduced us to a wonderful product called a Bumbo. It is a small booster chair made out of a low-density foam material. It helps align the baby's spine and has a front support that looks like the front of a horse saddle and helps prevent the baby from sliding forward. Julia absolutely loved it. I think she felt very independent sitting on her own and holding onto the front support. Ronan's head support is not as good as Julia's, but he did well with it also. We'll definitely be purchasing one soon.

It was fun to watch Samuel's development since he is only a few months older than the twins. It is kind of like the previews at the movies. Samuel can now sit up without assistance, and he has started to eat some solid food. He also giggles and laughs quite a bit. Right before they left, he was sitting next to Ronan, and he grabbed his head and pulled him close to snuggle. It was very sweet to watch.

I really enjoyed the social time with Amie too. It was nice having another adult around. The kids were on their best behavior. Amie and I decided that the kids get as tired of looking at us all day as we get tired of looking at them. They really like the chance to interact with other people. That is two lessons I've learned in the last two weeks. Not only do they appreciate a change in scenery, but they also appreciate a change in company. Fun six-month-olds are at the top of their list although the 2 ½-year old twins from last week were also entertaining.

February 6, 2007

We took the twins to visit a daycare today that we hope they will both be attending soon. Tender HealthCare specializes in "medically fragile" children. There are only twelve spots, and a ratio of one staff member for every three kids when there is full attendance. We were very impressed with the facility and program. They have nurses, therapists, and teachers who are wonderful. They have lots of activities including story time, singing, playing, pet therapy, arts and crafts, and cuddling. Ronan snuggled up to each staff member who held him.

The youngest child they have right now is a year old, so everyone was excited about the small babies. In addition, Julia's big blue eyes always get a lot of attention. They have one opening right now, and Ronan should be able to start in late February. They may have an opening in early April for Julia. We were impressed and thought the program will help the kids catch up with their peers. Daddy is taking a vacation day today so Mommy can have a bit of a break. We are looking forward to Grandma Gilda's visit on Sunday. She has offered to babysit for a few hours so we can have some time alone.

211 February 7, 2007

Photographer Aimee from Pure Expressions Photography came over to do a photo shoot of the kids today. This is a follow-up of the one she did in the NICU in September. Other than a short nap by Julia and a very dirty outfit by Ronan, everything went well. Julia slept through the first set of pictures. It turned out to be a good thing since when she woke up, she was quite perky and smiley. Ronan was wide-awake for the first set of pictures. He was looking all over the place, and it was hard to catch him in between movements.

Aimee shot some pictures of them alone and some of them together. I think she might have caught Ronan holding Julia's hand. When we moved downstairs, Julia woke up and was a complete ham for the camera. She was smiling up a storm and genuinely happy to be in this day. It was amazing to watch her. Ronan might have posed for a few smiley pictures too. Julia did some great tummy time shots and showed off how she can pull herself up. Ronan declined to do any tummy time shots so we let him off the hook. Thank you, Aimee—we had a great morning.

212 February 8, 2007

Julia had her physical therapy assessment today. She did very well. The physical therapist scored her within the normal baby curves for development of her motor skills and muscle development. In fact, the physical therapist told us that in twenty years she has only seen a handful of kids who were born this early score so high. Julia's only problem is her inability to turn her neck to the left when she is lying on her back. The physical therapist thinks it might be a habit she developed early on and recommended we try to entice her to look to the other side by waving toys. She said that she is not worried yet but will be if Julia does not improve in the next month. The occupational therapist at the hospital also recommended some exercises for her.

Ronan attended his Special Infant Care Clinic appointment today. His favorite occupational therapist, Lisa, examined him. She said he has made a lot of progress since he was in the hospital the last time. She said Ronan's reflux is severe and causes him a lot of discomfort, but she was pleased with the progress he has made with his tongue. We were instructed to continue giving him tummy time every day so he can strengthen his upper body and neck muscles.

We also stopped by the NICU for a visit with Nurse Dawn and NNPs Elizabeth and David. Everyone was very impressed with the amount of weight he has gained. He had a nice snuggle and short nap with Dawn. Elizabeth managed to pull him away from Dawn for a few minutes to have a short snuggle too. It is always nice to see old friends.

February 9, 2007

This morning Ronan went to the speech therapist. He had a very good session. She thought he did a lot better than he did last week. He took a record 90 ml from his bottle while working with her. The speech therapist also did some oral therapy with Ronan with a device called a Nuk. It looks like a toothbrush, but the end has a rounded massage brush with soft flanges on the top. She is trying to teach him to be more efficient with his sucking. He did very well with the Nuk but didn't like when she touched the insides of his cheeks with it.

Julia had a visit from Nurse Amy today. Julia was extremely sociable and, at one point, let out a long happy giggle. It was a nice surprise since we've only heard her do this a few times. She is such a happy baby. Julia is back to her regular feeding schedule after a few weeks of light eating. She will usually drink at least 120 ml at each feeding. However, today she drank 150 ml at two feedings. The last few nights, she has gone ten hours between feedings so we're glad she is trying to compensate during the day. Daddy is very happy that she has been sleeping through the night. Both kids are usually awake and smiling when we go into their room in the morning. It's nice to see Ronan enjoying life a bit.

The other exciting piece of news is that we got permission to go down 10 percent more on the calories in Ronan's TPN. We have a long way to go, but every step down is a step toward eliminating it.

This was a pretty good week. Scheduling activities every day really makes things more pleasant. It keeps the kids occupied and makes things more interesting for Mom. Things seem to be getting better overall. Julia is sleeping through the night and is happy during the day. Ronan has been in better spirits, too. His cranky time is much less frequent than it was when he first came home. He is gaining weight and making progress with his tongue. We are starting to decrease his TPN and increase his feedings.

February 13, 2007

Ronan had a fever again, and we had to take him to the hospital again. Fortunately, it was another false alarm, and he did not have an infection in his Broviac. While he was there, we convinced the GI doctors to give him a trial run without his TPN. He has been gaining so much weight; we think he might be ready to get along without it. He has two weeks without his TPN, and he has to prove to the doctors that he can gain weight without it. We have to weigh him every day and take him back to the GI doctor in a week. We're trying not to get too excited, but it would be so wonderful if this were permanent instead of temporary.

February 18, 2007

On Sunday, our local newspaper had a series of articles on premature birth. They interviewed a family with a former twenty-five weeker who stayed in the hospital about the same length of time that Ronan did. They also interviewed the family of a former twenty-three weeker (a lone surviving triplet) who stayed in the hospital for 146 days. The article stated that the preterm birth rate is very high in North Carolina at 14 percent. A report released last summer by the National Institute of Medicine said that in 2003, 12.5 percent of all births were premature, up from 9.6 percent in 1983. Each year, more than half a million babies, one in eight of all newborns, are born too early, the report said.

Articles continued in the editorial section centered on babies born at twenty-two to twenty-four weeks and discussed the medical costs, ethical questions, and emotional toll involved with preemies in need of intensive medical care. The parents of these babies are often asked to make very tough choices about whether to provide minimal care or whether to be more aggressive with the care when babies face problems such as mental retardation, blindness, deafness, cerebral palsy, or significant developmental problems. Sometimes treatment does not work and only causes further pain and suffering to these babies who are just not developed enough to survive. We are thankful that we never had to make that choice. At one point, the doctors did prepare us that we might have to make such a choice with Ronan. It was a choice no parent should have to make.

After a long eight months, our family is now complete. We know the next year will bring many changes, and we are confident the twins will eventually catch up to their peers.

Epilogue

On February 21 during a routine check by the home healthcare nurse, she determined that Ronan's Broviac was clotted off. Sometimes, when there is a problem flushing it, they can give him medicine to clear the blockage. They sent us to the hospital to try the medicine, but it did not work, so the Broviac needed to be removed.

They'd prefer not to remove it so soon because Ronan has not yet proven he can gain weight without the TPN. However, they don't have much of a choice, and they agreed to remove the Broviac and not reinsert another. This is really good news because he will no longer have a line in his chest that needs to be cared for; he will no longer receive the liver-compromising TPN, and he will no longer be at risk for infection. The surgery to remove the Broviac is painful because of the scar tissue that has built up around the line so they will sedate him and perform a fairly routine outpatient surgery. Ed and I hope he will continue to gain weight in the coming weeks, and we won't have to have any more discussion about inserting a new Broviac. Our next step is to work him off the continuous feedings and onto full bottle-feedings and get the g-tube removed. We anticipate this will take several months.

On February 26, Ronan started daycare. The occupational therapist evaluated him and expressed some concerns about his development. That is not altogether surprising considering how sick he has been. The good news is that the staff will work with him every day. We are so lucky to have found this daycare. We are even luckier they had a spot for Ronan.

Julia is still on oxygen. It is not uncommon for it to be difficult to get a child with chronic lung disease off the last whiff of oxygen. We think she's almost ready. There will be a spot opening up for her at daycare on April 2.

My favorite time to watch them is late at night when they are lying together in their crib. They are almost always touching in their sleep. Sometimes the gesture is as small as a tiny hand touching the other's head. Other times they hold hands or touch heads. They are definitely showing signs of that special twin bond you hear so much about.

I can imagine the four of us someday taking a lot of joy from driving out to an amusement park and riding the rollercoaster together.

REFERENCES

- The March of Dimes does not endorse any specific products or brands.
- The mention of Carepages in this book does not suggest any affiliation with CarePages or an endorsement of this book by Carepages.
- Bard Broviac is a registered trademark of C. R. Bard Inc. or an affiliate.
- Mic-Key is a registered trademark or trademark of Kimberly-Clark Worldwide Inc.
- Page 26: NEC Information Source, This information was provided by KidsHealth, one of the largest resources online for medically reviewed health information written for parents, kids, and teens. For more articles like this one, visit *www.KidsHealth.org* or *www.TeensHealth.org*, ©1995-2008. The Nemours Foundation. *http://www.kidshealth.org/parent/medical/digestive/nec.html*
- Page 27: IVH Information Source, written by Patricia Bromberger, MD, neonatologist, Kaiser Permanente and published by McKesson Provider Technologies, © 2008 RelayHealth and/or its affiliates. *http://www.med.umich.edu/1libr/pa/pa_ivh_hhg.htm*
- Page 35: Oxygen Desaturation Source, The University of Utah. *http://uuhsc.utah.edu/wcservices/nbicu/virtualtour/common_problems/apnea.html*
- Page 46: Total Parenteral Nutrition Source, National Library of Medicine, National Institute of Health, AHFS MedMaster(tm) Drug Information, American Society of Health-System Pharmacists (ASHP). *http://www.nlm.nih.gov/medlineplus/druginfo/medmaster/a601166.html*
- Page 58: Apnea Source, The University of Utah. *http://uuhsc.utah.edu/wcservices/nbicu/virtualtour/common_problems/apnea.html*
- Page 153: Persistent Pupillary Membrane Source, Gelatt, Kirk N. (ed.) (1999). *Veterinary Ophthalmology*, 3rd ed., Lippincott, Williams & Wilkins. *http://en.wikipedia.org/wiki/Pupillary_membranes*
- Page 173: *The News and Observer*. Sunday February 18, 2007; Preemies, Parents Endure Ordeal; Premature Births: When Babies Are Born Before 24 Weeks, Tough Decisions Await; How Far Should we go to Save a New Life?

Authors' Biography

Nicole and Ed have been married for 13 years. They reside in Cary, NC with their twins, Julia and Ronan, and their pet cockatiels, Alexander and Zebulon.

Nicole holds a BS from The University at Albany, an MBA from North Carolina State University, and is employed by a major financial services company.

Ed holds a BA from The University at Albany, and is employed by a major computer manufacturing and services company.